THE VALEDICTORIAN OF BEING DEAD

THE TRUE STORY OF DYING
TEN TIMES TO LIVE

HEATHER B. ARMSTRONG

GALLERY BOOKS

New York   London   Toronto   Sydney   New Delhi

G

Gallery Books
An Imprint of Simon & Schuster, Inc.
1230 Avenue of the Americas
New York, NY 10020

First Gallery Books hardcover edition April 2019

GALLERY BOOKS and colophon are registered
trademarks of Simon & Schuster, Inc.

For information about special discounts for bulk
purchases, please contact Simon & Schuster Special Sales
at 1-866-506-1949 or business@simonandschuster.com.

The Simon & Schuster Speakers Bureau can bring authors
to your live event. For more information or to book an event,
contact the Simon & Schuster Speakers Bureau at 1-866-248-3049
or visit our website at www.simonspeakers.com.

Interior design by Michelle Marchese

Manufactured in the United States of America

10   9   8   7   6   5   4   3   2   1

Library of Congress Cataloging-in-Publication Data
Names: Armstrong, Heather B., author.
Title: The valedictorian of being dead : the true story of dying ten times to
    live / Heather B. Armstrong.
Description: New York, NY : Gallery Books, an imprint of Simon & Schuster, Inc., 2019.
Identifiers: LCCN 2018050011 (print) | LCCN 2019000046 (ebook) |
    ISBN 9781501197062 (ebook) | ISBN 9781501197048 (hardcover) |
    ISBN 9781501197055 (trade pbk.)
Subjects: LCSH: Armstrong, Heather B.—Mental health. | Depression,
    Mental—Patients—United States—Biography. | Depression, Mental—Treatment.
Classification: LCC RC537 (ebook) | LCC RC537 .A744 2019 (print) | DDC 616.85/270092
    [B] —dc23
LC record available at https://urldefense.proofpoint.com/v2/url?u=https-3A__lccn.
loc.gov_2018050011&d=DwIFAg&c=jGUuvAdBXp_VqQ6t0yah2g&r=M40YuKx
7ONAd AyP8sLYy9FirEHXYcVB_44DYtjog4Z9S9Ao6mAi5Zj8gVWqQ2D
f&m=vt-JRY2v4BGvHwpjyTYALUvWluILBfFHj0N-zfvX17Y&s=I3dXu
2JVaC5RX6dTcr6n1jUQJ36SOBTQfACzasl9HdQ&e=

ISBN 978-1-5011-9704-8
ISBN 978-1-5011-9706-2 (ebook)

In loving memory of
Minnie Ann McGuire

CONTENTS

PROLOGUE

"MY MOTHER MARRIED SATAN, and when he's here next time you'll see *exactly* why she divorced him."

My words were a bit slurred—they often are when you're coming out of anesthesia—and I looked around the room to find my mother's face so I could nod furiously in her direction. I wanted her to confirm this statement of fact to the three nurses in the room. *They needed to know.* This was the most important thing we could possibly talk about right then. I was insistent that we discuss this, like I'd had a few too many bourbons at a party and was convinced that if I screamed, "BUT I AM NOT DRUNK!" people would stop dismissing me and say, "You know, if you'd only screamed that three times, I wouldn't have believed you. It was the *fourth* time that did it. That fourth time changed my mind."

Instead, she cleared her throat and asked how I was feeling. How the hell did she *think* I was feeling? I'd been almost brain-dead for fifteen minutes. I felt fantastic! When you want to be dead, there's nothing quite like being dead.

And boy, did I do dead well. Dr. Mickey would often tell my mother that of the three patients in this study so far, my brain went down and stayed down better than anyone else's. I didn't hear him tell her this—I was almost dead every time they had this conversation—but my mother would tell me about what would happen while I was gone, about the discussions she had with him concerning the history of depression in our family. When she told me about my dazzling performance, I reminded her that when I want to do something well, I become the valedictorian of doing that thing.

No one does dead better.

That wasn't the craziest thing I would say when coming out of anesthesia. Discussing my mother's doomed marriage to Satan was the topic I brought up after the seventh treatment. A little crazier than that was after the initial treatment—the first time in my life I had ever been under anesthesia. I angrily and breathlessly yelled, "The girls will miss their piano lesson!" My vision was blurry, and while trying to blink my way through it I could see the outline of at least five people in the room. They were strangers to me in that intoxicated state, and they were laughing at me.

That was the only time I had a dream while coming back from death, that first time. It was a very short dream, but its significance was not lost on me or my mother. My mother doesn't have much experience with angry drunks—she is an active Mormon who surrounds herself with other active, Diet Coke–drinking Mormons—but she immediately told the room that what I had uttered was very serious, that they should ease up on the laughter.

Dr. Mickey had told me during my consultation that it might take anywhere from twenty minutes to an hour to come out of the anesthesia, and in my dream it had taken so long that I was late to take my girls to their weekly piano lesson the following night. I was panic-stricken, seized with terror like I had been every afternoon for the previous six months when I would sit down to practice piano with my younger daughter. Marlo was seven at the time and had begun taking lessons in the fall of her second-grade school year. She had shown interest in music throughout her life and would dabble at the keys on our piano because her older sister Leta had been taking lessons for years.

I would never blame my wanting to be dead on my daughter's daily piano practice. It was a turning point in this eighteen-month-long bout of depression, but it was one of many. Each of them was in the downward direction. However, Marlo's ability to bruise her forehead on the keys of the treble clef took me down a few more notches than anything previous, past a point of no return. To a place in my closet where I would hide from the girls when I called my mother to scream. I tried so hard to conceal my pain from my children, and my closet was the most secluded space in the house. I always hoped that my clothes would muffle the sound. Sometimes I would scream words, and sometimes I would just let the sound of the pain erupt from my throat. (Imagine the noise a pig makes in a barn fire.) Sometimes after she said hello I would utter without any emotion, "I don't want to be alive anymore."

I had given my older daughter the gift of music in her life, the ability to read notes and play those notes on a piano. I wanted to give that same gift to Marlo; it only seemed fair. However, I don't play the piano very well, and her father, who is a classically trained pianist, had moved 2,200 miles across the country. The help I'd had when Leta learned to play piano was no longer available. Now, I'd been a full-time single mother working a full-time job for over three years.

It was up to me to get Marlo through her required practice every day. One more knife to juggle, and I was already juggling so many. My mother begged me to let it go, to look at the bigger picture and know that Marlo would lead a fulfilling life without piano.

But that wasn't a fair request. When you're depressed and no longer want to be alive, it's kind of impossible to let things go. Her father's leaving had left a gaping hole in Marlo's heart, and I didn't want to let his absence rob her of this as well. I wouldn't allow it. And in pursuit of that principle, I was willing to want to die.

Which is why my outburst of "The girls will miss their piano lesson!" hit my mother in that hospital room and almost knocked her against the wall. How appropriate that I would reference piano, That Which Made Me Want to Be Dead, while coming out of an experimental anesthetic procedure that would hopefully make me not want to be dead anymore. My mother shushed the room. She begged them not to laugh, remembering me begging on the phone, "Please, *please let me be dead*."

THE VALEDICTORIAN OF BEING DEAD

ONE

CALLING ALL ANGELS

ONE MONTH BEFORE MY first treatment, I had a face-to-face appointment with my psychiatrist. He required this before he would agree to refill my medication. Normally, his secretary would call my pharmacy when I needed more Valium or Neurontin or Trazodone, but I had not been in to see him in over nine months. I'd been busy, I told him, when he asked why I hadn't made an appointment. That's the answer I give to every single person who cannot possibly comprehend what day-to-day life is like for a full-time single mother who also has to work full-time. "I cannot get coffee with you, sorry. I cannot have lunch with you, I cannot go to book club, I cannot volunteer at the second grade Halloween party. I'm busy; incomprehensibly, bafflingly busy."

Turns out, though, that "I've been busy" is not a good enough answer for Dr. Lowry Bushnell, the head of the electroconvulsive therapy (ECT) clinic at University Neuropsychiatric Institute (UNI) on the campus of the University of Utah. I was sitting across the room from him, my body an upright corpse, when he set down his notepad with a thud and cocked his jaw angrily to the side. He explained that the longer you let a depressive episode go untreated, the harder it is to climb out of the hole. He was mad at me and shook his head. How could I have let this go on so long? Why had I waited over a year to seek his help? Why hadn't I called him when the symptoms of my depression reappeared?

The answer to those questions was long and complicated, so I summed it up with one sentence: "My ex-husband will try to take away my kids if he knows I'm this depressed."

I had finally said those words out loud to someone who wasn't my mother or talk-therapist, and usually when I said them to my mother I was screaming. Every moment of the morning routine and the afternoon routine and the bedtime routine and All of the Things Needing to Get Done was haunted by the memory of the very real threat he'd made to take away my kids. My "ongoing suicidal ideation," he said, made me an unfit mother, but before he could argue that in front of anyone with the authority to strip me of custody, he moved to New York. I'd managed to balance raising two young girls alone while running a full-time business for over three years. I imagine that anyone who does this has once or twice or many, many times thought, *It would be nice if I didn't wake up tomorrow.* Not because we're suicidal or want to kill ourselves. We know that's not an option. We'd never do that to our children. We just want a break, and sometimes the desperation for that break is terrifyingly bleak.

"It doesn't matter what your ex-husband will do if he finds out, Heather, especially if you're dead. He'd certainly find out then!" Dr. Bushnell said. I hadn't told him that I'd very much like to be dead. Medical professionals have certain obligations when it comes to hearing that word and words like it from a patient's mouth, and

I didn't want to end up unwillingly committed to any sort of facility. But I didn't have to say it.

"I would ask you how you're feeling, except you don't have to tell me," he said. "It's all over your face. It has stolen your eyes."

Suddenly he got up from his seat and walked over to his desk to pick up his phone. He brought it back with him to sit across from me once more and said, "I have an idea and I want you to consider something." I remained perfectly still as he called his colleague, Dr. Brian Mickey, to see if he was looking for any more patients to participate in the experimental study he was conducting at the ECT clinic. Dr. Mickey was investigating an alternative to electroconvulsive therapy that may have fewer side effects that result from the electrically induced seizure at the core of that procedure. He had heard about a study conducted in Austria in the early 1990s that used the anesthesia isoflurane to mimic ECT. Dr. Mickey's study, however, would be the first ever to use propofol anesthesia, a less intense drug.

With this treatment, Dr. Bushnell explained, a patient is simply put to sleep with the intravenous anesthetic approximately three times per week for ten treatment sessions. The study is designed to determine if "burst suppression"—quieting the brain's electrical activity—can alleviate the symptoms of depression. "Quieting" here is the polite way of saying "taking down to zero" or "almost braindead." Dr. Bushnell likes to call it "a really deep induced coma that makes you feel better about yourself." The anesthesiologists called it "the abyss."

"She's sitting in my office right now, yes," Dr. Bushnell told Dr. Mickey. "Good, then. I'll let her know all of that." He talked me through the details of the study after hanging up the phone and asked if I would consider looking over the official paperwork.

"You're the *perfect* candidate for this study, Heather," Dr. Bushnell said. "You have a history of depression. Your family has a history of depression. This latest bout of depression has lasted more than a year. You're young and healthy and . . ." He then paused and moved toward the edge of his seat and put his hands on his knees. ". . . and most importantly, *I know it will work*."

I left his office with a handful of papers, including a release form I would eventually sign. It ensured that the hospital and those working on the study would not be held responsible if I suffered any of the side effects possible from dying ten times. This treatment would take place just down the hall from Dr. Bushnell's office in the ECT clinic on the south side of UNI, a building that sits on a winding road called Colorow Way. I drove out of that parking lot and headed to the grocery store to buy two gold Mylar balloons—a giant number 1 and a giant number 3—for Leta, who was turning thirteen years old that day. I was hosting four of her friends for a sleepover and thought the balloons would complement the festive atmosphere.

"I didn't realize how big the numbers would be once they were filled with helium," I said to the woman helping me with my order. I wondered how in the hell I was going to fit these things into my car while processing everything Dr. Bushnell had just told me.

"No one does!" she said as she tied off the end of the number 1.

"I'm going to walk out of here with the numbers reversed so that people will think I'm turning thirty-one," I said, "because I could totally pass for a decade younger." I made a dramatic sweeping motion with my hand from my head to my torso, as if presenting a great beauty wearing a tattered gray hoodie, black yoga pants that had been slept in the night before, and hair that had not been washed in six days.

"Honey," she shot back as she filled the number 3, "I'm pushing sixty, so I only wish I looked as good as you."

After she tied a ribbon to the end of each balloon, I paid and attempted to wrangle the enormous numbers as elegantly as possible. They filled the entire backseat of my SUV, and I had to adjust the rearview mirror and stick my head out of the window in order to maneuver my way out of the parking lot. *My daughter is becoming a teenager today,* I thought. *If I hit anyone or anything, they'll have to forgive me.* When I successfully pulled out of the strip mall, I breathed a heavy sigh of relief and could feel myself smiling.

Twenty minutes later I arrived home and texted my mother and asked if she could talk. This is how my mother and I communicate, and it is the only acceptable way of calling someone on the phone today. Yes, I grew up in a home that had only one landline and routinely beat my fists on my older sister's bedroom door, the coiled cord of the phone strung taut underneath it. Thankfully, we no longer have to live through that kind of hell. She immediately texted back, "I can." I wondered how many texts I had from my mother from the previous eighteen months that said exactly that.

"I just joked around with an employee at the grocery store," I blurted after my mom said hello. "I just found myself doing it; it just felt normal and easy. I can't remember the last time I did that. I interacted with a stranger and smiled at a stranger. I can't remember the last time I *wanted* to do that."

When I wasn't in my closet screaming into the phone about my desire to be dead—whenever I was having a calm or technical call with my mother, I would walk around the living room in a giant circle. As I passed by the piano for the third time, I started to cry and she asked if I was okay. And I was. I was okay. Actually, I was more than okay. I was okay and yet simultaneously torn. It was this tension that made my eyes fill with tears. Because of course I would be the one in the family who is so crazy that she has to get some scary procedure done in a hospital. And not just any hospital: a procedure done at *that* clinic. You know the one. Where they shock people because of their *mental disorders*.

Of course I am the craziest one in the family. The black sheep. The one who left the Mormon faith and registered Democrat. The fuckup.

And yet . . . for the first time in over a year I felt hope. I felt like maybe I wouldn't feel like this forever. I'd been certain I would live the rest of my life wanting to be dead. I had resigned myself to wanting to be dead. But what if it didn't have to be that way? What if what Dr. Bushnell said was true? What if this treatment worked?

"Let's do this," my mom interrupted my winding stream of thoughts, to assure me that we were in this together. Her words were firm and forceful and conclusive.

"But you will have to drive—"

"I don't care what I have to do. I will fly to the damn moon and back if I have to. *We're doing this.*"

What I explained to my mother about the procedure was only what my psychiatrist had explained to me. Even though she said she didn't need the details, I asked her to listen to me talk through it so that I could gain confidence in the hope that I felt.

First, I'd had to meet a relatively rigid set of requirements in order to qualify for the treatment. I couldn't be suffering from an addiction or a personality disorder. I couldn't be experiencing a manic episode. I had to have been going through a bout of depression as severe as mine for over a year, and it had to have been treatment-resistant depression. My depression qualified, as my antidepressants had stopped working after twelve years and a few modifications made a year prior had produced no positive effects. Yes, I could still fall asleep at night, but my meds had stopped enabling my ability to cope with life. Second, ECT has proven to be the most effective way to combat treatment-resistant depression, although other chemicals such as ketamine have been used to some good effect as well. ECT works by shocking the brain and producing a seizure. This seizure causes the brain to flatline temporarily, and it is this flatline that some believe is the benefit of the entire apparatus. It's like rebooting a computer. And anyone who has ever had problems with a computer knows that sometimes you have to turn it off and on again several times to fix whatever glitch was causing all your applications to crash. This is why most patients undergoing ECT endure anywhere from ten to twelve treatments. Each time the brain is reset, it gets a little better. Third, previous studies using an anesthetic called isoflurane had shown significant promise, although that drug was difficult to recover from and caused dysphoria in many of the patients. It almost always caused nausea as well. Dr. Mickey had tried to get a more controlled and randomized study funded for isoflurane, but when that failed, he had to come up with something more novel and interesting. And because both propofol and isoflurane can induce a burst suppression state in the brain, he picked up the idea for a propofol study and managed to push it through. Propofol as an anesthetic had proven far easier on surgical patients than isoflurane. All of this is why I agreed to ten rounds of Dying in Front of My Mom.

I wouldn't find out until several months later that after my mother hung up the phone she fell limp into my stepfather's arms and wept. She sobbed because she'd heard the hope in my voice. To her it sounded like the angels she was calling upon every night in her prayers. And she'd continue to call upon them until treatment began four long weeks later.

"And this . . . you see this vial?" It was my first treatment, and the anesthesiologist was trying to explain exactly what would happen and

why. Today it was Dr. Tadler—there would be five different anesthesiologists in total—and I appreciated that he was being so thorough.
I nodded, because my anxiety in that moment had stripped me of my
ability to speak. In subsequent treatments he would touch my arm. I
needed that warmth of reassurance, because I was terrified. On the
paperwork I had signed, one of the possible side effects listed was death:

RISKS:

Very Rare (less than 1/10,000): Complications including life-
threatening cardiac arrhythmias (irregular heartbeats), respiratory
arrest (inability to breathe), myocardial infarction (heart attack),
stroke, and even death are possible.

Even though I wanted to be dead, I needed to get my kids to
piano practice the following night. If I died, they would be late.

"This is fentanyl—it's an opiate—and we give you this just in
case you get a headache when you come out of the propofol, which is
in this one." He then held up a much larger vial filled with a milky-
white substance. A nurse and Dr. Mickey's research assistant both
affixed a single wire to my forehead with Velcro squares. I felt the
small pinch of each hook of fabric attaching itself to my skin. I would
often wonder in the drunken state that followed each treatment how
a piece of Velcro could stick to my forehead if my forehead was not
made out of the other fabric that makes Velcro *Velcro*.

The nurse checked one more time to make sure that the tube connected to each drug was firmly inside the 22-gauge needle they'd placed
in my vein thirty minutes before and taped taut against the skin of my
arm. God, that needle. The *whole process* of that needle. I've never had
a hard time seeing blood or having my blood drawn, and have bragged
about this skill to each and every phlebotomist in my medical history.

"Don't even look; just jab that spike right in there. Seriously, I won't even flinch." But then, I'd never met a needle like this needle. When I saw it for the first time, I remembered the scene in *Jaws* when Roy Scheider's character catches his first close-up glimpse of the shark.

"You're gonna need a bigger boat."

I had my right arm laid out on a thin table separating me from Molly, the phlebotomist for my first treatment, who was filling out my drug history on a computer screen. We'd chatted quite a bit as she gathered all the materials she'd need to insert the needle, and there were many.

I bragged about being the valedictorian of having my blood drawn and explained that after giving birth to Marlo without any pain medication, I didn't really have a hard time with running headfirst into a brick wall. She nodded and shared her birth stories with me, one in which she barely made it to the hospital in time for someone to catch her son as he shot out of the birth canal like a cannon. I tend to find my tribe very quickly: I can immediately sense whether my brand of humor is going to make someone feel at ease or run away in horror. Molly was the former, so of course I told her that the doctor who delivered my second daughter had never before presided over an unmedicated birth and was so mystified by the experience that she jabbered endless, fascinated nonsense as she was stitching up my vagina. My doula had to stop her and say, "Let's save this conversation for later."

We were shaking our heads over each other's stories when she said that she needed to go over my list of medications and ask when I had last taken each one.

"We're going to be here all day," I warned her.

She pulled up my history on the computer and scrolled from the top all the way to the bottom. After what felt like hours of scrolling, pursing her lips, and nodding, she said, "This is not the absolute worst I have seen." My tribe.

Before each treatment—before they inserted the needle, even—each phlebotomist had to go through this list.

"This one?" they'd ask.

"Last night," I'd answer.

"This one?"

"Last night."

"This one?"

"Last night."

Back and forth until . . . oh, wait, it's still going on. We haven't made it to the end of the list yet.

The only medication I take that isn't for depression and anxiety is a drug called Macrobid, because I inherited a urinary tract whose shape makes it prone to infection after sexual intercourse.

I received no sexual education in my Mormon upbringing. Not a word of advice or warning, no tips. *Tips*, ha! Even those will give me a urinary tract infection. *It is that bad.* I got a UTI the first time I ever had sex, because no one ever told me, "You must go pee after intercourse, so make sure you head onto the court with a full bladder and a toilet nearby."

The full-bladder strategy worked for me for a few years, until it didn't and I had to start showering immediately after sex. Then I had a baby, and now screw all your strategies and pointers. Peeing doesn't work, showering doesn't work, and I don't want to hear any cranberry juice nonsense. Through no effort on my own part, I have become the valedictorian of being resistant to every DIY approach of curing a UTI. I brag about this on my résumé. Now I must take an antibiotic after I have sex, every single time. Just one—thankfully, not a full course—that is specifically engineered to attack bacteria located in the urinary tract.

When Molly got to the Macrobid on the list, she had to say it a few times to get the pronunciation right.

"Macro-bid," I said, to help her along.

"Oh, okay. Macrobid," she said, and continued, "When was the last time you took this one?"

"Hahahaha!" I just laughed and laughed, and because she made me feel so at ease, I thought she deserved an explanation. "I only take that drug after I have sex. It prevents me from getting a UTI."

"So . . ."

"A really, really, really long time ago. It's not in my system anymore. Maybe I should take it for all the bats flying around in my vagina."

Molly was my phlebotomist four more times, and every time that she'd get to the Macrobid, I'd interrupt her and say, "Still housing bats, Molly. Still."

I'm glad she was the first one to attempt the needle—the *whole process* of the needle. Apparently the gauge of this needle was far bigger than the other needle they use for ECT procedures. Because I was only the third patient to enter this study, she and everyone else were having to get used to the difference. Every maneuver leading up to inserting the needle was exactly the same as what happens when I get my blood drawn, right down to the part where I point my head toward several bulging veins on the inside of my elbow and say, "I have been told by several practicing doctors that I'd be very good at taking heroin."

Molly nodded, thanked me for making her job easier, and then tapped on a blue vein that had become as round as my pinky finger because of the tourniquet she'd fastened near my shoulder. And then she plunged the needle into my arm. I probably should have warned you about that sentence in case you are uneasy with the idea or talk of needles and blood. But, you see, it was just as sudden and unsettling for me. I was forbidden to eat food in the sixteen to eighteen hours leading up to a treatment and had to stop drinking water several hours before. I would show up each time famished and dehydrated—so dehydrated, in fact, that I was a phlebotomist's worst nightmare. This could potentially ruin my résumé, especially since I am usually the valedictorian of remaining hydrated.

I go everywhere with a water bottle. If I were to go outside and peer into my car right now, I bet there would be at least five water bottles scattered across the front seat, occupying every cup holder in the center console and in the doors—water bottles I have put there just in case I make a trip to the grocery store and they've run out of water.

Molly would have to try at least five times to get that thing in my arm. It did not want to enter a vein, not even the one that had grown at that point to the circumference of a grape. It was uncomfortable and awkward. It felt like someone jammed a tree trunk up into my shoulder via my elbow, hooked up my humerus to an electrical socket, and was flipping it on and off. When she finally did get it in—not just the tip, the whole thing—she was panting and sweating, and I was woozy.

———

My mother said that she always knew the instant the propofol would take effect. I have vague memories of clenching my hands near each other at the top of my chest as everyone was assembling the equipment—the vials, tubes, wires—and this clenching of my hands has always been a barometer of my anxiety. When I suffered postpartum depression with my first daughter, I would find myself sitting on the floor in the corner of my room when she was napping, my hands clinched into fists that I'd tuck up under my chin. Many times I would be unable to unclench them, and I'd use my mouth and teeth to pry each finger open so that I could flatten out my hands and use them to push my body up off of the floor. Afterward I'd have red indentations from my incisors on each finger.

Since I was lying flat on my back on a gurney with a needle and a series of tubes hooked into my arm, I couldn't get my hands all the way up underneath my chin, where I would have preferred them. At home, I usually ran to the couch or my bed and curled into the fetal position, my clenched hands taking their place under my chin. If I was not at my house, I'd run to my car and crawl into the back seat, shove Marlo's booster chair onto the floor, and tuck myself into a ball with my back facing outward in case anyone walked by to find a woman in her car having a panic attack. If they could see my face, they would see the terror; so I reasoned that if they saw the back of my head, they would assume I was taking a nap. In my car. In the parking lot of the grocery store.

I had to tuck my hands on my chest because of all the appara-tus, and my mother said that my fists were so taut, she thought my knuckles might break through my skin. I was anxious, scared, and frightened—but not of dying. I was not afraid that they would be unable to bring me out of the anesthesia. I was terrified that I would never stop feeling this way—that I would always want to be dead. I could remember a time when I didn't feel this way, *but I couldn't remember what that felt like*.

When the propofol hit, my mother would watch my fists come undone, a cascade of skinny fingers, and my hands would fall to the gurney with a soft thud. It was an immediate physical manifestation of the drug doing what it was supposed to. My mother knew this; she'd seen other people undergo anesthesia before. But not like this—not for the purpose of making someone almost brain-dead. Not for the purpose of making *her daughter* almost brain-dead.

The first time, not even a minute after they had shown me the vials of fentanyl and propofol, something went terribly wrong. The nurse had just finished affixing the Velcro shapes to my forehead and I remember someone saying that I should soon feel the fentanyl taking effect. Dr. Tadler had just touched my arm, and the warmth of his hand still lingered there. But suddenly every form and line and figure in the room started melting. The walls dripped like wax and coagulated on the floor. Heads and arms and torsos turned into jagged crayon cartoons. Noses and hair grew into triangular knives. Someone's mouth stretched across the room and laughed, and teeth big as tree trunks grazed my face.

"Something is wrong! Something is wrong!" I screamed, but the fentanyl was taking effect and my scream came out only as a whisper. My mother said she could tell something wasn't right before I coughed out those words. The look of fear already on my face had turned into horror. I closed my eyes so that I wouldn't have to witness the bodies dissolving around me. And then . . . *nothing*. There was a brief blink of nothing, a blip of total darkness, and then I realized I was taking too long to come out of anesthesia. I only had thirty-six hours to get my girls to their piano lesson, and this was taking too long. Someone needed to tell the doctor to hurry or we were going to be late. *Please, someone tell him*. The piano teacher's face appeared, disembodied and transparent. I could see the wall of the hospital room through her forehead and cheeks. I thought of the scene from *The Wizard of Oz* when Dorothy's house is caught inside the tornado, and people and animals float by outside her window— one by one—and you can see the tornado behind them. The piano teacher was as concerned as Auntie Em, wondering where I was. Why wasn't I on my way? I'd never been late before, and I couldn't get the words out of my mouth to tell her I was trying. *I was trying.*

I thought that if I blinked a few times that her face might become less transparent, that she'd be able to see me better, so that's what I tried. I blinked and blinked. But her face disappeared and the wall behind her forehead turned into the shapes of people. Two in front of me. I blinked again. One to the right, two to the left. Where was the piano teacher? I couldn't find her. I blinked until finally my tongue could articulate a consonant.

"The girls will miss their piano lesson!"

They immediately wheeled the gurney into a room directly adjacent to the one I'd been in for what they called a recovery period. They would hand me a cup of apple juice and ask me a list of questions. I remember being so thirsty that I guzzled the apple juice like I was chugging a beer and then drunkenly demanded, "Another!"

"Can you tell me your name?" someone asked me—someone I had not seen or met before. He had not been in the room during my treatment.

"Who are you?" I shot back, but not because I was mad. I was startled and drunk and didn't know why a strange person had appeared like magic.

"I'm Chris. I work here in the recovery room," he answered. "Can you tell me who you are? Your full name?"

"I'm *Heather B. Armstrong*," I answered.

"Excellent. Now can you tell me what year it is?" he asked.

"Nineteen seventy-nine," I answered.

"Nineteen-what?"

"*Seventy-nine,*" I said slowly and condescendingly.

"Could it possibly be another year? Can you think a little more about it?"

Everyone looked at everyone else. I really, really hate it when people do this. I get angry because it makes me paranoid, like I'm not in on the joke. Or maybe everyone knows the building is about to blow up and they don't want to alarm me.

"It's not 1979, is it?" I asked, since my mother was not backing me up. She had looked at my stepfather, who looked back at her. The two of them would be with me at every treatment. They would sacrifice a minimum of eight hours a day, three times a week, for three weeks so that I could participate in this study. One of the rules for participation, in addition to fasting for a minimum of twelve to eighteen hours beforehand, was having someone drive me home. This is normal for any sort of surgical or anesthetic procedure: drunk people aren't supposed to operate heavy machinery. But I had to undergo ten treatments. I would need someone ten times: two times the first week, three times each during weeks two and three, and two times the final week. That's a lot of times. That's like handing someone your baby and saying, "Here, hold this for one second while I tie my shoe," and then disappearing forever.

What makes this even more complicated is that I never knew what time I'd go in for a treatment until the afternoon before. It varied depending on how many patients they had coming in for ECT. Since mine was an experimental study—and since we never knew if it would take twenty minutes or an hour for me to wake up—I had to be either the first or the last patient of the day. Only once did I have to go in at 7:20 a.m. as the first patient, and that was for my first treatment. My mother and stepfather were supposed to pick me up at 7:00 a.m. Instead, they showed up at 5:45 a.m., before my alarm had gone off. They are habitually early to everything.

My siblings and I always joke about this.

"Mom says we're meeting at your place at five p.m.?"

"Yeah, between five and five thirty p.m. is good."

"Which means Mom will be there—"

"At noon. She will be here at noon."

She's a good sport when we joke about it in front of her. You have to be a good sport in my family, because we show love by making fun of each other. That sounds terrible, but it means that we are comfortable enough with each other to show that we've been paying enough attention to learn our quirks and to celebrate how wonderfully funny those quirks are. If we're annoyed by a quirk, we don't make fun of it. No, we just stew in judgmental resentment until it festers into an ulcer and we end up at the ER. One time my brother had to spend three days in the hospital because my dad refused to tip a server more than five percent at a Chili's.

In ten out of ten treatments I never got the date right. Not once. When I woke up from the anesthesia and they asked me my name, I aced the test all ten times. But each time they asked what year it was, I answered 1979 or 2012. One of these two specific years, and I'd be insistent about it. Every time. If my mother is ever in the room when I'm writing a check, she now has every right to say, "You do know that a bank is not going to cash anything written in the seventies."

hand wrapped around my thigh so that it wouldn't clench itself into a fist I'd be unable to release.

"Where are you? Where are the girls?" she'd ask, always trying to hide the sound of dread in her voice.

"They're asleep. They can't hear me. I can't do this, Mom. *I only have two hands! I only have two hands!*" Then she'd let me cry. She would sit on the other end of the phone and let me pour the misery out of my body in howling electric waves. I cried a lot by myself, too—I cried every day. I cried every time I took a shower and hoped the warm water on my face might calm the swelling underneath my eyes—that is, on the rare occasion that I took a shower. I often couldn't find the energy to shower, change my clothes, or brush my hair.

"But you will feel so much better if you take a shower," people often told me. I wanted to tell them that this is not something you say to a person who wants to be dead, even if you mean well. I've taken showers—hundreds if not thousands of showers—in my life. I know what a shower is like. Showers did not ever wash away this feeling. In fact, I would have to stand there and brace for the jolt of the first splash of water against my skin. That piercing change of state—going from dry to wet in less than a second—felt like jumper cables had been attached to every nerve in my body. Not only was I alive, I was alive and *wet*. I understood why cats sometimes maul their owners during a bath.

That same change in state, but now reversed when I stepped out of the shower—from hot to unbearably cold—was so overpowering that I'd have to steady myself against the sink to keep myself from collapsing to the floor. The air around me was heavy enough on its own, and suddenly I was carrying the weight of the water in my hair. When I dried my face, I'd see that the temperature of the water had been no match for the inflammation under my eyes, and I would

TWO

I ONLY HAVE TWO HANDS

WHEN MY MOTHER AND stepfather woke me up before my alarm on the morning of my first treatment, we immediately tried to figure out the logistics of the next two hours of our lives. I suggested that my stepfather accompany me in my car, drop me off, and then go back to the house so that he and my mother could get the girls ready for school. This all seems way too complicated when I try to explain it, and it *was* complicated. The timing of my first treatment completely disrupted my morning routine with my girls, a routine as regimented as any program in the armed forces. It had to be.

"I only have two hands!" I had sobbed this to my mother on the phone almost every night for over eighteen months. Sometimes I'd be in my closet so that my hanging clothes would absorb the sound of my agonizing crying and the girls wouldn't hear. Sometimes I would escape to the other side of the house and find a dark corner where I could call her and hold the phone with one hand, my other

think of the excuses I would give to everyone who would see me that day and ask, "What happened? Are you okay?"

The answers varied depending on the person.

"Yeah, I'm fine. I just had a long night."

"It's been a really long week is all."

"Kids, you know. I was up all night."

"I'm okay. I just need to get some sleep."

I also hated any confrontation with my naked body, so I often wore the same clothes three days in a row. I lived in yoga pants, sports bras, and T-shirts. When I spilled coffee or food on my shirt I'd use a baby wipe to dab the stain and clean myself. If crumbs fell out of my mouth, I'd wipe them straight to the floor. That's why I had a dog.

I didn't understand what had happened to my body in such a short period of time, why I would look down at my stomach and legs and see a strange, unfamiliar figure. I hated seeing myself naked. I am tall and thin, but every inch of my body was bloated and deformed. The water in the shower intensified the curves of these foreign bulges, and as a form of self-torture I would grab a wad of flesh between my fingers and shake it up and down, like I was jolting it awake, telling it to go home.

My belly made me the most uncomfortable, and it's why I couldn't wear most of my normal clothes anymore. Nothing fit. Every pair of jeans throttled the tops of my hips like it was choking a neck it had once kissed, once draped with a loving arm. The bloating was so pronounced that I could slouch at a certain angle while standing up and make myself look pregnant.

I didn't share this part of my depression with everyone, because I didn't want to hear the yammering body image lecture. The response would be "But, Heather, you could stand to gain ten pounds." Or: "But, Heather, if you gained ten pounds, no one would even be able to tell!"

I could tell.

People would tell me to embrace my body and all of its imper-fections. I would have to, there in the depths of the worst depression of my life, tell them to shut up on behalf of every other person, big and small, who doesn't want to take a shower and see their own naked body. I would reconsider body image and what it means to have a healthy sense of my physical self when I no longer wanted to be dead, if that ever happened.

My body did not feel like my body, and every movement I made reminded me of this. Every time I reached for the handle of the re-frigerator to grab the milk for the kids' cereal in the morning, I could feel the inside of my arm graze my side. And it did not feel like my arm. It did not feel like my side. These were not my shapes and lines and curves, and every time I reached for the milk, I thought about it.

Every time I moved my body, I thought about it. Every time I breathed, I thought about it. When your body doesn't feel like your body, you're allowed to have an emotion about it. You can't help but experience an emotion about it. And no emotion is right or wrong, especially if it is visceral. My emotion tangled itself inside every joint of my body so that each time I bent a leg or scratched an itch, I could feel it shrieking.

I had not had these thoughts plague me for over twenty years. Back then, instead of just walking around in the same clothes for three or four or six straight days to deal with it, I would starve myself. And when the starvation became unbearable, I'd finally give in, eat 3,000 calories in less than ten minutes, and immediately make myself puke.

My sister has a completely different body type from me, and yet. We heard the same words come out of our father's mouth *time and time and time and time and time again* when we were kids: "This is what a beautiful woman looks like." He'd be pointing to a voluptuous blond actress on the television or a petite yet busty model on the cover of a magazine. A beautiful woman was round in all the right places and tiny everywhere else. We both looked at ourselves and did not see what he was describing at all. We were not beautiful. My sister was curvy but not thin and wanted to look like me. I was thin but not curvy and wanted to look like her. I at least got to experience a twenty-year reprieve from the constant *thinking about it*, but my sister? I don't think she's ever been free of it for a full second of her life. And I can hear people now if they were to see my stunningly gorgeous sister, if they knew she had those thoughts, the "Oh my God, what is she thinking? But she's so beautiful! She should own her curves!" Bullshit, bullshit, bullshit.

On her behalf and that of every other woman who *cannot stop thinking about it*, I will get on with this story, but not before asking you to please stop. Just stop it. We will get there in our own time, and if we never do, we never do.

———

The morning routine was the easiest routine we had, my two daughters and I, even though it was the one I dreaded the most. Because it began with waking up and realizing I was alive. Again! Jesus Christ, *it just kept happening*.

The moment my alarm would go off I would shoot straight up and gasp for breath as my anxiety set fire to every molecule in my body. I tried so many times to explain this sensation to people: what an instantaneous rush of anxiety feels like first thing in the morning. It's very different from its more jovial counterpart, the panic attack. My mother would often ask me if it had happened again, and I always answered yes, that I woke up soaking in a vat of acid, that my flesh was covered in flames. The thought of what I needed to get done and what I hadn't gotten done and every potential thing that would ever need to be done screamed in my ears, voices all talking over each other in angry, disappointed tones, all echoing and thundering and crashing into cymbals.

I'd hit SNOOZE so that I could compose myself for All the Things Needing to Get Done and lie back on my pillow, my hands curling into fists and making their way up under my chin. I would be able to feel my heartbeat throbbing in my neck, set to whatever acceler-ated rhythm my anxiety had chosen that morning. Often I tried to swallow over and over again to force myself to calm my breathing.

After lying there for three snoozes—twenty-seven minutes—I would turn off my alarm, pull my body up, and drape my legs over the side of the bed. When I turned on the lamp beside me, I would look down at my black yoga pants, which were wet from sweat. I slept in my yoga pants because I didn't want to feel sheets or blankets against my flesh. I didn't want to look at my bare skin in the morning. I didn't want to have to change my pants and see my alien body. People often joked with me that they would love to work from home all day like me, since they wouldn't have to put on any pants. But guess what? We have it so easy that we don't even have to take them off in the first place. We can sleep in what we wore yesterday and wake up really upset that we're still alive.

I would then drag myself out of bed and head downstairs to feed and let out Coco, my miniature Australian shepherd, who was nine years old at the time. I love her, but she barks and howls and is so fiercely protective of my children that she has several times slipped through a brief opening in the front door to chase and scare the literal shit out of someone who just happens to be out for a jog. She sleeps in a crate for her own safety—so that I don't murder her.

Every morning, without fail, she would howl as she ran upstairs to get her breakfast. She'd howl and spin like a whirling dervish while I screamed, "STOP IT! STOP IT! STOP IT!" I would go straight from soaking in a sweat bath to trying to wrangle a Tasmanian devil flipping over herself to get to her bowl of food, the sound reverberating through the house like shattering glass.

I then headed into Leta's room to wake her, and even in the weeks and months when my anxiety and depression were at their worst I still cherished the delicate silence. It was dark in there, and because she sleeps spread out like a windmill I never knew which body part was where. I never once sat down on her mattress as intended because a limb would be wherever I tried to put my body. I'd learned to sit gently, slowly, and brush my hand over her forehead if I could find it. If I couldn't, which was often, I would just rub my hand back and forth over the blanket wrapped four times around her body. She'd eventually rouse, and neither of us said good morning, and I liked that. I liked that she said, "I'll meet you in the kitchen?" with a question mark. She knew she had a few more delicious minutes to sleep, since I had to wake Marlo.

I'd leave Leta's not-question question and walk into Marlo's room, and because my eyes were now more adjusted to the darkness, I could see where to place my body on her bed. She is a fellow windmill sleeper, and since her bed was so close to the ground, I often found her splayed like a starfish facedown on the floor.

And it could have been due to Marlo's age—no, I don't believe that for a second; I do believe it has everything to do with Marlo's personality—that I had no idea what I was gonna get. Sometimes she'd be a totally gentle snuggle bunny and immediately wrap her arms around my neck so that I could pull her up from the mattress and carry her from her room to the kitchen. She was growing into the long limbs we'd given to her as lanky parents, and whenever I got to hold her like this, I'd nestle my head into her neck underneath a braid of her hair and think, *Remember this. Remember this. Remember this.* Remember when she used to call her morning waffle "bref-disk" through her chipped front tooth.

Remember baby hobo-bobo Marlo, who may or may not have gotten ringworm on her face from sucking on the dog's ears—hold on to *that* Marlo—because many times she woke up with a directive from the universe: *Burn it to the ground.* She never woke up in an instant fit of rage. No, the rage would build slowly, in waves.

Leta would hear us heading toward the kitchen and stumble out of her bedroom, sometimes awake enough to look at me like "Which Marlo did we get today?" I would always nod, no matter which card we happened to pull, just to acknowledge that I was bracing for it, too. The rumbling would begin when she pulled the stool out from underneath the countertop and angrily set down the blanket she'd brought with her to bref-disk across the seat. Like *This again! This whole sitting here having to eat food prepared by my loving mother again? Burn it to the ground!*

Sometimes she'd climb up into the seat, pull the blanket around her, and just stare into space. Sometimes she would put her head down on the countertop and cover her ears as if the conversation I was having with Leta about spoons was just too stupid. Sometimes she'd answer me when I asked if she wanted a waffle or a bowl of cereal, and this was when we really knew just how violent her rage would be. Either she'd eat her meal in absolute silence or she'd eat her meal while telling Leta in great detail how everything she was doing now and the night before was totally and completely wrong. And then they'd begin to argue.

Leta is five years older than her sister and should know better than to defend herself. Marlo wanted Leta to defend herself so that she could say, "Oh, look. You're wrong there, too." This bickering noise was a trigger for me, especially in the morning when I was trying to make sure we got everyone out of the door on time, and to quell it I would set down the knife I was using to spread chocolate across a piece of white bread with crusts cut off. (This "sandwich" was the only thing I ever packed in Marlo's lunch that I knew for certain would not return home uneaten.) I'd tell Leta in front of Marlo, "You do realize she's baiting you. You are a little fish looking for a worm and she just reeled you in."

"But she just told me that I'm chewing with my mouth open, and I'm not! I'M NOT!" And I understood. I know what it's like to be deliberately misinterpreted, to have someone say that I am doing one thing when in reality I am doing just the opposite.

"We both know you are not. *You* know that you are not. That's all that matters." And then I'd tell them both to hurry up as I finished stuffing Goldfish crackers, flavored cartoon fruit snacks, and a small container of seedless grapes into Marlo's lunch.

One of my biggest accomplishments as a parent—I will brag about this long before I ever bring up stellar report cards—was getting my kids to put their dirty dishes where they were supposed to go. It was not easy, but now, not two hundred years after I first started nagging them, my children will finish a meal and ask, "Sink or dishwasher, Mom?"

If the dishwasher is full of clean dishes, it's the sink. If I haven't run the dishwasher, it's the dishwasher. Simple, sure. *But I did that.* My kids are polite and say hello and goodbye and thank you and please. They stand up for the misunderstood kids in their classes. They go to bed when it's time to go to bed. And they put their dishes where they are supposed to go. There is not a nature-versus-nurture argument to be made here, because I did that.

This all may not sound like a chaotic routine, and that's because it isn't by design. I did this by myself morning after morning after morning, and I made it this way. I braid both of my girls' hair the night before so that they don't wake up with tumbleweeds on the tops of their heads. Both girls are able to dress themselves, and I don't care if Marlo looks like she has chosen her wardrobe while tripping balls. If she will be warm when she needs to be warm or cool when she needs to be cool, I do not give one whit what she wears. This is a battle I chose not to fight because for far too long I had to fight Marlo to put on *any* clothes. And any clothes are better than Naked Seven-Year-Old Shows Up for Second-Grade Math.

And that's the thing: I have never sent my kids to school naked. I never have! They show up on time if not early. They have their supplies, their lunch boxes, the homework I had to sign. Their hair is brushed; their teeth are clean. They wear coats when it's freezing outside. They've recently had showers and baths, and the one who should be wearing deodorant is doing so. Leta says she loves me at least five times as she's walking out the door to catch her carpool; she loves me, she thanks me for everything, she can't wait to see me this afternoon. And Marlo and I walk hand in hand to the long hallway at the front of her school to wait for the morning bell. I rub her tiny knuckles with my giant fingers when we head toward her class—*Remember this*—and I wait next to her doorway as she puts her things into her locker across the hall. She looks over her shoulder at least three times to make sure I'm still standing there—I always am—and when she's finished she comes to me, wraps her arms around my waist, and squeezes as hard as her little limbs can. I squeeze her back, careful not to crush her, and then she holds out her hand so that I can put a kiss in her palm—a kiss she will hold in her fist and press against her face whenever she's feeling lonely or frustrated.

I do a really fantastic job. I'm good at this; anyone who has as much practice as I do would be good at this. And I only have two hands. How had I just done it again? How would I possibly do it again tomorrow? I did a great job of disguising the agonizing monotony: *Make sure they've eaten, make sure they're dressed, they've showered, make sure they have all their homework. Is Marlo wearing socks? Make sure to remember to call the office and tell the secretary that Marlo has a doctor's appointment in two days. Make sure to let the dog back in. Where is the dog? Make sure we have enough Cheerios for the next two breakfasts. Make sure I signed the permission slip. Make sure Leta has taken a pill for her allergies; make sure Leta has asked her friend for a ride to school tomorrow, since the other carpool just canceled. Make sure to tell them, "Sink!" because the dishwasher is full of clean dishes.*

Morning after morning after morning. And then again. And then again.

No one knew that I wanted to be dead. That's how good I am.

But then, as I'm driving back to the house to begin working, still dressed in the same clothes I've worn three days in a row, I suddenly remember, *Oh no!* Marlo was supposed to have taken empty milk cartons to school for an art project, and I totally forgot. She will be devastated—she always is when I forget this kind of thing—so I really try to stay on top of it. I should be *better* about staying on top of it. And I will think of this exact moment when I wake up the following morning in a vat of sweat. I will hear through the howling Satanic chorus of All the Things Needing to Get Done—that low whisper, now becoming a roar, that she would be so much better off without me. Someone else would have remembered those milk cartons. Someone else would have collected them weeks ago. Someone else would have spared her that sadness. Someone else would be a better mother.

They would be so much better off without me.

THREE
THE MICHAEL JACKSON DRUG

AFTER MY THIRD CUP of apple juice and several minutes of awkward silence and knowing, concerned glances passed around the room, I suddenly blurted, "It's 2017!" The year finally emerged in my brain—a brain that had just exhibited no activity for over fifteen minutes—like a word you've been searching for that suddenly comes to you two days later when you're enjoying a completely unrelated hamburger. I could hear my mother's shoulders relaxing, and I would later learn that her sigh of relief was so heavy because I didn't wake up from the anesthesia for almost two hours. Add the stress of that to the idea that I might not remember the last thirty-eight years of my life, and the Mormon God would have forgiven her if she had taken me home and immediately raided my liquor cabinet. He would have lit her a cigarette.

I repeated my name and the correct year a few more times before Chris asked me if I thought I felt strong enough to swing my legs over the side of the gurney. All I could think about was the chocolate protein bar I had stashed in my purse.

I knew I was going to be ravenous after fasting for so long—I hadn't eaten anything in over eighteen hours—so I told Chris I was fine and not to worry about me. Nothing to see here. I swiftly draped my legs over the gurney and didn't even wait for anyone to ask me if I thought I was able to stand up on my own. I just did it, and that's when the headache almost knocked me to the ground. A searing bolt of electricity shot through my head from my left temple to my right, and it blinded me for several terrifying seconds. I couldn't see. I couldn't hear. I could only feel a thundering throb of pain through every corner of my head. I frantically grabbed at my ears and tore at my hair, an involuntary reaction that removed my hands from the gurney beneath me. When I began to sway underneath the weight of the pain, my stepfather reached out to steady me, a gesture that would be only one of countless ways in which this man helped save me.

I had not been able to remember the correct calendar year after coming out of anesthesia, but I clearly remembered Dr. Tadler telling me beforehand that they were giving me fentanyl to prevent any potential headaches from the propofol.

"You mean the Michael Jackson drug?"

"Yes, the Michael Jackson drug."

"The drug that killed Michael Jackson?"

"Yes, that one."

"But that's the drug that killed Michael Jackson."

"I just told you that, yes."

I had this conversation over and over again when I told anyone about the treatment and was always tempted to moonwalk while answering the first question.

I remained in my stepfather's embrace until I regained my sight, although the pain at that point had become so rhythmic in its throbbing, it resembled a low, driving bassline. Once I was able to demonstrate that I could walk a few feet, they let my parents escort me out of the building to their minivan. When my stepfather opened the giant sliding door to the back, I dove in head first, quite literally, over the seat and into my giant purse. I found that protein bar and wrapped my fingers around it so tightly that I almost crushed it.

After wrangling my body into the seat so that my stepfather could shut the door to the minivan, I slouched with the entire weight of my body on the armrest in the center of the back seat. Air felt heavy on my face and chest, and even moving my arms was tiring. I don't know how I got the protein bar out of its packaging; my mother probably helped after noticing my entire body lolling. Suddenly it was in my mouth and I experienced a brief two-second respite from the agony of my headache.

The back windows of my parents' minivan are tinted, something I only just then noticed.

I noticed the tint on the windows only because the sunlight in Utah at that time of year hit at an uncomfortable, punishing angle, and the tint did nothing to shield it. My headache had begun to pulse in sync with my heartbeat—it had traveled down the side of my forehead and settled into the back of my jaw where I could feel it in my teeth—and the rays of the sun were crushing my skull. I tore at my head again and finally rested both of my arms over my face to block out the light.

"You should get the tint on these windows fixed," I mumbled through the headache. "The tint doesn't work. Who makes a tint that doesn't work?" It's always odd, the things over which we obsess when we are tipsy or, as in this case, totally wasted. I was dealing with the headache that normally follows a bender, mixed with the agony of a high that has gone horribly wrong and has you pleading for it to end.

"Someone, please make it stop," I moaned again and again. We wound our way down 900 South, past the park and into my neighborhood. Every right and left turn would swing the pain in my head in lurching diagonal lines. When we pulled into my driveway, I waited for my stepfather to open the minivan's sliding door, having no strength to do it myself. He helped me walk to my front door and from there I held on to the walls and the countertop in the kitchen to steady myself. I finally made it to the staircase that led into my basement, down into my dark, cavernous bedroom with blackout shades hanging in the windows. The wooden railing guided each torturous step toward the welcoming black clutches of sleep. As I fell onto my bed and pulled a pillow over my head, that punishing, lying voice of despair spoke over the drumming vibration of my headache: *This isn't going to work. This isn't going to work. This isn't going to work.*

They would be so much better off without me.

FOUR

JUST HOW BADLY DO YOU WANT TO BE DEAD

"YOU'LL TELL THEM I can't take the fentanyl, right? Please? You'll tell them? Because I can't do this if it's going to be like this every time. You'll tell them?"

"Of course I'll tell them," my mother assured me from the front seat of the minivan, the three of us together again, winding up 900 North toward the ECT clinic. Today I'd have my second treatment, and the afternoon before they had called to tell me to come in at noon. I had stopped eating the night before at 7:00 p.m. and had my last gulp of water before I fell asleep at 11:00. My stomach was rumbling and gurgling, mostly from hunger, but also from anxiety. Yet another lovely side effect of my constant state of panic was what I called the Anxiety Shits. You didn't want to know this about me, but then I've already told you about the unique shape of my urinary tract.

It was a good thing that I hadn't had a bite of food that morning, otherwise I'd have spent every ten minutes running in and out of the bathroom. When faced with a deadline or when Marlo would whine about practicing piano or when adding yet more items to the list of All the Things Needing to Get Done, my anxiety would not only begin to choke me, it would defeat my body's ability to handle food. I'd get diarrhea as bad as that which I once suffered after eating raw fish in Peru.

Oddly, I had missed something crucial during the first treatment. They were also giving me Zofran to combat possible nausea. Fentanyl, propofol, *and* Zofran, which I would later find out can cause constipation in certain people. You'll never guess who is one of those people.

When we pulled into the parking lot at the south side of UNI, I asked my mother again, "You're going to tell them, aren't you?" I couldn't—no, I *wouldn't*—continue with the treatment if what had happened the first time was going to be how I lived my life for the next month. I didn't ever again want to experience a hallucination like the one I had experienced while going under. When I woke up from my headache nap that afternoon, I felt hungover and *irritated* in every part of my body. I don't know what other word to use to describe the sensation. I didn't get a moment of relief until I climbed back into bed that night—after the homework routine, after piano practice, after putting my shoes back on and driving to my child's middle school to watch her sing as part of an ensemble chorus in a full production of *Chitty Chitty Bang Bang.*

My gut was telling me that whatever had happened concerned that vial of fentanyl. It's a powerful opioid, and after the birth of both of my children I illegally gave away all my hydrocodone and oxycodone to friends, because those drugs make me violently ill. This was before I knew that the opioid crisis is an actual crisis. The day that I brought Marlo home from the hospital, I took a hydrocodone for the pain of having pushed an eight-pound baby out of my body, only to start vomiting so ferociously that I ripped my stitches.

We entered the clinic and the sterile smell hit my face like a cold, wet rag. That sounds unpleasant, but it wasn't terrible. It smelled like winter—frosty and aseptic, different from the smell of a normal hospital, where the smell of disease seems to hang in the air. A long corridor connected the front doors to the waiting room where I had to check in. They'd ask me my name and date of birth more than once and wrap around my wrist an identity bracelet. Usually a guy named Greg sat at the check-in desk. He was a little shorter than me and had thick, dark hair and a matching mustache. He wore a different pair of sneakers every time I saw him—hip sneakers for millennials, although he didn't strike me as being that young. He radiated an air of being completely comfortable in his own skin, the kind of confidence you earn through years and years of life beating you over the head. I always wanted it to be Greg at the desk. He never asked too many questions and always smiled and said hello so genuinely that I instantly felt like I had known him my entire life.

"Everything's good, so just fill out the sheet and I'll go see when they're ready for you," he said, handing me a clipboard with a double-sided piece of paper hooked to the top. Before each treatment I had to fill out a questionnaire titled "The Quick Inventory of Depressive Symptomatology (16-Item) (Self-Report) (QUIDS-SR 16)" or what I liked to call "16 Ways to Determine Just How Badly You Want to Be Dead." I'd check one response next to each item that best described how I felt for the last seven days.

Each item indicated a symptom of depression and the responses were graded 0, 1, 2, or 3.

1. **Falling Asleep**

0   I never take longer than 30 minutes to fall asleep.

1   I take at least 30 minutes to fall asleep, less than half the time.

2   I take at least 30 minutes to fall asleep, more than half the time.

3   I take more than 60 minutes to fall asleep, more than half the time.

Falling asleep wasn't ever a problem for me, not with the amount and combination of medication I took each night. I wondered if my answer to this question alone would downplay the seriousness with which I did not want to be alive. Thirteen years previously my psychiatrist treated me for postpartum depression during a four-day stint at UNI. I had not slept for more than thirty minutes at a time for over six months. He prescribed a mixture of drugs that essentially cured my insomnia even though his intention was to treat my anxiety, a wonderful by-product that I had now enjoyed for over a decade. In fact, if I know I am going to be on the phone with someone close to my bedtime, I will wait to take my medication until after we have spoken. Otherwise I might fall asleep mid-sentence.

I took great relief with the second item, though, because surely they'd see my answer and think, *okay, we get it now*.

2. **Sleep During the Night**

0   I do not wake up at night.

1   I have a restless, light sleep with a few brief awakenings each night.

2   I wake up at least once a night, but I go back to sleep easily.

3   I awaken more than once a night and stay awake for 20 minutes or more, more than half the time.

This would be the second time I would mark a thick X in the box next to 3 and underline the whole sentence four times. I even put a few exclamation points next to the box. I never had a problem *falling* asleep, but rarely did I ever sleep through the night. Much of my anxiety toward the end of each day centered on the fear that I'd wake up at one or two o'clock in the morning and be unable to fall back asleep for two or three hours. Once I was awake, I was awake. I was awake in a state of total panic thinking about how impossible it would be to get everything done: piano lessons, piano practice, deadlines, dance lessons, therapy, math homework, dentist appointments, parent-teacher conferences, laundry, grocery shopping, meal making, dog walking, dish washing, bill paying, meetings, conference calls, deadlines, deadlines, deadlines.

If by chance I did fall back asleep, I'd be restless until my alarm would go off and cue the routine: shoot straight up and gasp for breath as my anxiety set fire to every molecule in my body. I had come to dread nighttime again like I had during my postpartum depression when I would wonder about the baby, *Will she sleep tonight? Will she sleep tonight?* But instead the refrain had become, *Will I sleep tonight? Will I sleep tonight?* "Wonder" isn't the right word to describe how those questions sounded in my brain. I wasn't *wondering* about it. Those repeated worries appeared as faceless apparitions tucked into a dark corner of my head, their arms wrapped around their torsos as they rocked back and forth.

The next item on the Quick Inventory was "Waking Up Too Early." If by "waking up too early" you mean 2:00 a.m., then yes. Next, "Sleeping Too Much." The nap I had taken after the first treatment was the first nap I had taken in over a year. In college, when my depression was just the good old-fashioned, generic, run-of-the-mill, I-hate-myself depression, sleep was my only escape. I could nap through a Category 5 hurricane. But having kids turned my depression on its head, and now it manifests as anxiety, and napping is a distant memory. I have friends who talk about growing up with depressed parents who experienced episodes so bad that they wouldn't get out of bed in the morning. When my children grow up, they will tell their friends about the year I walked over 20,000 steps a day. Sitting still is for people who can cope.

The fifth item was "Feeling Sad," and again I underlined and circled and almost ripped a hole in the paper next to box 3, which said, "I feel sad nearly all of the time." I couldn't remember what it felt like to be happy or even fine. I would have gladly taken fine, because "fine" would mean that I wouldn't live the rest of my life wanting to be dead. How many times in the months leading up to this treatment had I asked my mother and my therapist, "What if this is it? What if this is the nervous breakdown that people have, the one they don't recover from? What if this is my final nervous breakdown?" How many times had I pleaded with them both, as if they could in any way honor my request, "Please, *just let me be dead.*" If I were dead, I wouldn't be sad all the time.

Items six and seven asked about appetite, whether I'd experienced an increase or a decrease. When I saw items eight and nine, again I almost ripped up the paper.

8. **Decreased Weight (Within the Last 2 Weeks)**

9. **Increased Weight (Within the Last 2 Weeks)**

Could we please not bring up my weight? Every time I moved my body, *I thought about it.* Every time I breathed, *I thought about it.* I'd lived over twenty years of my life free from the torture of thinking about it, but I couldn't remember what that felt like. *What would it be like to* not *think about my weight?* How amazing would it be to free up that brain space?

Item 10 concerned concentration and decision-making, and here again I did not fit the mold of traditional depression. I put an X in the box next to 0, which said, "There is no change in my usual capacity to concentrate or make decisions." I'm good at this. I do a really fantastic job managing all of this: Imagine me waving my arms around in wild circles to indicate ALL OF THE GODDAMN THINGS. Indecision is not an option. Struggling to focus is not an option.

And then came item 11. Oof. A punch in the gut that knocked the wind out of me. Again.

11. View of Myself

0   I see myself as equally worthwhile and deserving as other people.

1   I am more self-blaming than usual.

2   I largely believe that I cause problems for others.

3   I think almost constantly about major and minor defects in myself.

I wasn't allowed to choose more than one response, but I wanted to check 1, 2, and 3. They were all true. I immediately thought about the morning I had forgotten to send empty milk cartons to school with Marlo, or the times I had run out of the room away from the piano because her refusal to practice was making me angry to the point of tears. All the pain I had caused my mother and stepfather, how many times they made the forty-minute drive from their home to mine because I had cried into the phone about *laundry*. Sure, I did a really fantastic job managing all of this, but I hated myself for the way I *felt* about it. I hated that I dreaded waking up. I hated that I dreaded going to sleep. I hated that I cried all the damn time. I hated that Leta would see the panic in my eyes every morning and ask, "Are you okay?" knowing that I wasn't okay. And more than anything else I felt foolish. I felt like an idiot that I hadn't anticipated the choices and sacrifices I would have to make for my kids in order to be able to raise them alone and what that would do to my full-time work, what juggling all of it would do to my career. I was a failure. I was a fraud. I was less than that.

I was nobody.

12. Thoughts of Death or Suicide

I checked the box next to 1: "I feel that life is empty or wonder if it's worth living." The other options did not apply to how I felt about being alive. I didn't have plans to kill myself nor had I ever tried. I didn't think of suicide. I did not daydream of ways I would end my life. I just didn't want to be alive. Daydreams consisted of eternal blackness and silence, an end to the hamster wheel of my day-to-day existence. I daydreamed about the annihilation of my senses—an end to the feeling of dread. Death would extinguish the fire inside my chest and brain. Yet, I did not ever consider specific ways I would try to make that happen.

But make no mistake: I wanted to be dead. I yearned to be dead. *Please, let me be dead.*

13. General Interest

Was I interested in people or activities? I easily checked the box next to 3: "I have virtually no interest in formerly pursued activities." And then I scribbled "Or people" in the margin.

The woman who filled Leta's Mylar balloons was the first stranger I had willingly interacted with in months. When going about my life in public places, I avoided eye contact and either nodded or shook my head in response to questions, even if those questions warranted more than a yes or a no. I didn't want to risk getting into a conversation with someone, didn't want to exchange words because of the pain of existence. That sounds so dramatic, and I'm guilty of having such tendencies. But this was just the opposite. Words held drama and theatrics and *meaning*, and I wanted no part of it, especially with a stranger.

And as for activities? Was this a joke? My day started and ended with no break in between. I imagined what it would be like to flip through a home decor magazine and pause to admire a set of striped pillow shams. Or sign up for a cooking class. Or grab lunch with a friend.

The final three items asked me to consider the physical manifestations of my depression: "Energy Level," "Feeling Slowed Down," and "Feeling Restless." I hadn't ever thought about my energy level. It hadn't ever occurred to me to consider it.

My God, I certainly didn't feel slowed down. Feeling restless? *Of course* I felt restless. *Of course* I could barely stay seated and needed to pace around, and 20,000 steps a day were not going to walk themselves. The dishes were not going to wash themselves. My sick kid was not going to drive herself home from school and bring herself a bowl in which to puke.

As I filled out the questionnaire, my mother found a nurse and asked if she could relay a message to Dr. Mickey. Just as I was signing my name to the bottom of the paper, he walked into the waiting room and took a seat across from the three of us. His boyish blond hair bounced with every movement.

"Seems you had a reaction to something last time?" he asked, leaning forward, his arms perched on his knees. I nodded and told him about the horrifying hallucination I'd had before going under—how I'd battled a headache that entire afternoon and evening—and mentioned that I'd had adverse reactions to opioids in the past.

"A hallucination . . . Have you ever had a hallucination with an opioid?"

"No," I answered. "But they nauseate me, and I have never understood why someone would want to abuse a substance that makes you feel like you're in your first trimester of pregnancy."

He grinned. "I'm not quite sure what that feels like, but we can certainly leave out the fentanyl this time and see if it makes a difference. It's not critical to the study. We're just trying to *prevent* a potential headache, and it looks like we failed miserably."

Dr. Mickey wore thick black glasses and dressed in neatly pressed pants and a tie. He stood a few inches shorter than I did and always spoke softly but deliberately. During the initial intake interview he had run through a list of questions about my history with depression and the current episode I was suffering. The question I remember most was the last one: "Do you feel like you have a reason to live?"

I couldn't look at him and instead stared at my entwined fingers resting in my lap. The tears involuntarily started pouring down my face and onto the scarf I'd worn that day to hide the dirty shirt underneath it. I didn't say a word and barely shook my head. He set down the pen he'd been using to comment on my answers. Then he paused before saying, "You have so much to live for, and you deserve to feel that way. It must feel horrible that you don't."

FIVE

NO MEMORIES, NO DREAMS, NO LIGHT AT THE OTHER END

MOLLY WAS NOT MY phlebotomist for my second treatment, and I had no rapport with the woman who was desperately trying to get that needle into my arm. We'd gone over my list of drugs and the last time I'd taken each one and she'd collected all the gear she would need to insert the needle. After four unsuccessful attempts on my left arm, she started to ask if she could try a vein in my right, even though that was the arm where the needle had been inserted for the previous treatment. Their plan was to switch arms each time to give each one a break, but I interrupted her question to scream, "YES!" I startled myself, even, with the desperation in my response, but she had just spent over five minutes torturing me with a 22-gauge needle.

The needle went smoothly and directly into the same vein from the previous treatment, and she taped the end of it down so that it lay flat on my forearm. I walked back into the waiting room and took the seat next to my mother.

A nurse I had not seen before then walked in and motioned for me to follow him. They were ready for me, and the three of us followed him directly across the hall into the room where my gurney sat in the middle of the floor dressed in off-white linens. The anesthesiologist—someone other than Dr. Tadler—was gathering materials, and Dr. Mickey and his assistant were looking over some paperwork. I passed by the nurse, who asked me to confirm my name and date of birth and to take my place lying down on my back. The nurse asked if I'd like a warm blanket and this would become one of my favorite parts of dying, of going down to zero, slipping away into nothingness: the warm hospital blanket. He pulled one out of what looked like a refrigerator, except its shelves were lined with blankets like the one he very sweetly spread from my feet up to my neck and helped tuck between my arms and torso. It was as if he was telling me with that gesture that he knew this was scary—they all did—but he cared enough to offer me something as intimate as warmth.

Another nurse I hadn't seen when I walked in worked with Dr. Mickey's assistant to prepare the Velcro attachments that they then affixed to my non-Velcro forehead. I will never understand the science of that.

Everyone worked quickly and seamlessly, a choreography of human hands in rhythm. Without getting up from his stool, the anesthesiologist wheeled himself over to introduce himself. The comfort in that elegant dance calmed me and my parents. My stepfather was seated next to the doorway, my mother was walking back and forth in front of him. She wasn't pacing, she was getting her steps in for the day: 20,000 at a minimum so that she would not only keep up with me on our Fitbit trackers but also *beat* me. I don't get from just anyone my drive to be the valedictorian of everything.

"I'm Dr. Larson and I'll be the one working with you today. It's really nice to meet you," he said, and offered his hand. Both of my hands had already assumed their clenched positions on my chest, but I managed to release my right hand and take his in a brief exchange.

"You're in charge of the propofol today," I said back flatly. "The drug that killed Michael Jackson."

"HAY-THER!" my mother called from the end of the gurney.

Dr. Larson laughed and said, "Well, you could put it that way.

"Dr. Mickey said that you possibly had a reaction to the fentanyl last time. We're going to look into that, and thank you for telling us so that we can modify this for you and possibly for future participants. Again, we're going to give you Zofran for possible nausea, propofol, and a different, less powerful drug. When the anesthesia enters your arm, it can sting, and the fentanyl was supposed to help with that, too. We're going to give you just a bit of lidocaine. Have you ever had that drug? Maybe at the dentist's?"

Why, yes, I had been given lidocaine many times at the dentist's. *And it was glorious.* I had no idea that I'd enjoy that numb feeling in my lips and gums as much as I did, and I'm not even sure why I did other than to guess that, God, isn't it great when you don't have to feel anything?

"I know what lidocaine is, yes," I said to Dr. Larson. "And if you have any extra, could you also numb my mouth?" My mother just glared at me. "Don't look at me like that, Mom," I said as they connected the vials to the needle in my arm. "If I die, that will be the last memory that I have of you."

But there were no memories. No dreams. No tunnels leading to a light at the other end. No visions. When Dr. Larson told me that he was starting the propofol, I looked up to find Dr. Mickey's face, his gentle eyes, and wondered if I was powerful enough to resist the anesthesia. How long could I stay awake? Could I fight it for seconds? Minutes? What if I could fight it for—

And then nothing.

Since I'd been under anesthesia only once, I didn't know if what I experienced was like what other people experience when they go under. Maybe people who meditate have taught themselves to envision nothing when they close their eyes, but my mind usually darts in and out of images of All the Things Needing to Get Done. But the black nothingness of a really deep coma—like, all the way to zero—was like having all my senses shut off with a switch. A black curtain descended and smothered me, swallowed me whole. No color, no smell, no texture.

I never remembered closing my eyes, never remembered the moment the anesthesia would devour me. But my mother would tell me two weeks later in a fit of tears—it would take her two weeks to be able to talk about what she had witnessed—that I would go under so fast and so hard that they would race to get the giant spatula-shaped breathing tube into my mouth and down my throat.

"You were a rag doll. They handled you like a rag doll, sometimes more than one of them. They were racing against time, and sometimes it took more than one person to maneuver you. Your body had no life; your arms and head hung like limp wet rags as they struggled to get the tube in fast enough. I was certain you were dead."

Technically, I was. At least, my brain was. And Dr. Mickey would keep my brain in that state for over fifteen minutes, until he was satisfied with the length and movement of the lines on the monitor connected to the wire on my forehead. One line measured my brain activity; the other measured how much anesthesia they were administering. One line started at the top of the screen; the other sat directly opposite it at the very bottom. They would immediately beeline across each other to occupy the other side—a straight line at the bottom tracing the abyss—until it was time to bring me up and out of the nothingness, the lines sulking back to their original positions and creating a lopsided U with their paths. These lines, however, weren't nearly as important as the burst suppression ratio that they were measuring with the line at the bottom. Under certain kinds of anesthesia and when the anesthetic state is deep enough, the brain can experience a very unique bistable state: it's either flat and very suppressed or there's bursting activity. It alternates between these two states—between several seconds or even a minute of being very flat and quiet, there is a sudden burst, only for it to become quiet again—and the ratio between these two states was their ultimate goal. They were shooting for an 80 percent suppression rate for fifteen minutes. My mother said she'd often hold my hand when the lines sat at opposite ends, but I don't remember. I don't remember Dr. Larson removing the breathing tube from my throat and mouth. I don't remember taking the first breath by myself or the nurse wheeling my gurney into the recovery room.

I heard someone say something—I don't know who and I don't know what they said—and then I blinked my eyes open. They had propped up the top end of the gurney so that I was no longer lying flat on my back. I glanced around to figure out where the hell I was. I saw my mother and stepfather sitting to the left of the gurney. Chris, the recovery nurse from my first treatment, stood to my right.

"Nobody melted!" I suddenly realized, out loud. I turned my head to look Chris straight in the face and opened my eyes as wide as I could stretch them to emphasize this very important truth. "The people stayed people," I continued, except I was slurring my words and it sounded more like "The pee-poo stay pee-poo."

"That's really good to hear," he said generously, given that he almost certainly had no idea what I was referring to. "Can you tell me your name?"

I held up my arm and pointed to the bracelet Greg had affixed to my wrist when I checked in. "Heather B. Armstrong. With the *B*. Always with the *B*." He started to ask me the next question but I interrupted him with "Don't you know who I am?"—thinking I was being terribly funny when instead I was being terribly drunk.

"Yes, we all know who you are." These nurses are so used to hanging out with drunk people. "Can you tell me what year it is?"

"It's 1979," I answered. Again. My stepfather started to laugh, and I saw my mother reach over to put her hand on his arm, an indication to him that drunk people sometimes get really sensitive when they think you're laughing at them, although she was on the verge of giggling herself.

Chris cleared his throat and asked again, "Can you think a little harder about that? What year is it?"

I didn't want to think harder about what I knew to be true, so I blurted, "It's 1979." And as that number tumbled out of my mouth, a wall calendar appeared in my head, its pages flipping as if caught in a gust of wind—1985, 1993, 1997, 2001, 2004, 2009—until the whole daydream stopped at 2017.

"Oh yeah. It's 2017. Now I remember."

"Good," he said. "Would you like something to dri—"

"APPLE JUICE!"

I gulped two cups and listened to my mother describe the shape of the lines on the monitor. She gestured wildly with her arms and hands, although I was having a hard time concentrating in my drowsy, drunken state. Couldn't we talk about this later, maybe after a nap? I mean, I knew I'd just woken up, but being brain-dead for fifteen minutes is hard work, and I was the best at it. I had a reputation to uphold and wanted nothing more than to go back to sleep—a very different state from my usual panicking and pacing and screaming into the phone about laundry.

After a few more minutes, Chris asked if I thought I was able to stand up. I was so distracted by the unfamiliar state of fatigue that I wouldn't even realize until hours later—after attacking two chocolate protein bars; after the drive down 900 South in the back of the minivan; after a ninety-minute nap made possible because my parents had stayed after driving me home to watch my kids—that I didn't have a headache. In fact, *nothing* hurt save for the gaping puncture wound in my right arm.

I'd been right about the fentanyl.

The following week Dr. Mickey and Dr. Larson would tell us that they had to do an unforeseen amount of research into the matter, but turns out I can count myself among maybe four percent of the population of the entire world whose reaction to an opioid in the structural class of fentanyl could include the kind of delusions or hallucinations I'd experienced. The headache afterward was a bonus, a slightly more common side effect.

Not only was I the valedictorian of being dead, I was also the valedictorian of teaching these doctors new things.

SIX

MARATHON TRAINING FOR BEGINNERS

NINE MONTHS BEFORE STARTING this treatment, I made an appointment to see my talk therapist. I had not seen her in over a year. I hadn't needed to sit across from her and comb through my neuroses like I had every week for almost a decade when married to my ex. But my primary care physician didn't have an opening for a physical for another four weeks, and something was wrong. My body and mind didn't feel normal; they did not feel like my own. I needed to get some blood work done, maybe have my thyroid checked. I needed an official diagnosis—something to hold on to.

Melissa—or Mel, as she likes to be called—had moved her office to the fifth floor of a building close to downtown and had changed all the furniture. I felt a little disoriented when I sat down across from her on a sprawling leather sofa and picked at the tassels of an orange wool blanket draped over its arm. I began to speak and she interrupted me to say, "That is the stupidest thing I have ever heard."

"But I got to run the Boston Marathon! I mean, who—"

"Heather, are you a runner?"

"Well, sort of. I ran the New York City Marathon in 2011—terribly. I mean, I broke my foot—"

"HEATHER."

We'd always had this rapport, this dynamic where I was the china shop and she was the bull running wild. This was why I trusted her so much. She wasn't afraid to call bullshit, and she always set meaningful goals for our time and work together. Which was why I hadn't seen her in over a year. I'd met a goal we'd set together: I ended a three-year relationship that had gone on three years too long. He and I started seeing each other a few months after I separated from my ex, and I loved that man, I really did. But his jealousy was so all-consuming that he once accused me of having rough sex with another man because of the indentations left on my butt from sitting on a metal picnic bench. I can laugh about it now, but at the time he was stalking all of my social media feeds, cross-referencing them with my friends' social media feeds, and making an inventory of all the inconsistencies to prove: one, that I was lying about everything; two, that I didn't want to be in a relationship with him; and three, that I wanted to have rough metal picnic bench sex with someone else.

It had been two months since I'd run the Boston Marathon as a guide for a runner who was visually impaired. Mel literally fell out of her chair when I told her that detail. What on earth was I doing guiding *anyone*, much less someone who was visually impaired in a sport that I hate? But this is the one character trait I have that brings me as much joy as it does pain. When presented with an opportunity to suck the marrow out of life, I always say yes.

I'd said yes when someone from the Massachusetts Association for the Blind and Visually Impaired emailed me and asked if I'd be interested in this once-in-a lifetime opportunity. And *come on*, it's not like I would ever qualify to run the Boston Marathon. I'm an incredibly slow runner, not to mention that I hate running. It is my least favorite thing in the world. But, you know, the *Boston Marathon*. I remember thinking, *When I die, I will get to say that I ran the Boston Marathon,* having no idea that this very endeavor would be the thing that triggered the beginning of a depressive episode so horrible that I would very much want to be dead.

I can point to the day that I downloaded a Hal Higdon marathon training program for beginners, one that I printed out and pinned to the wall next to my desk, and say, "This is when it all went to shit." I always thought that one of the worst parts about being depressed is not knowing why. We never choose to feel this way. We'd give anything not to feel this way. And the most maddening thing we try to explain to people is that we know there is no reason for us to feel this way.

But then I found myself in a state of hopeless despair—*and I knew why*. And the knowing why didn't make it any better. In fact, I thought I'd stop being depressed once I'd finished the race. When that didn't happen—when the loneliness and feeling of desperate isolation continued to consume me—I wished that I hadn't ever had a reason to hold on to in the first place. Because what was there to hold on to now?

Also, telling people "I ran a marathon and it made me depressed" is not how anyone should ever talk about depression to someone who doesn't understand depression. I am passing that knowledge on to you in case you're terrible at running and get invited to guide a runner who is visually impaired in a marathon.

I even tiptoed around this when recounting it to Mel, and her profession requires her to understand the hows and whys and whens of depression. Because, yes, it was the physical act of running, but it was also what the running required of me, what it took from me, what it didn't give back. The training program for beginners totally works—it prepared me for the 26.2 miles of pavement between Hopkinton and Copley Square—but it was grueling and relentless and unforgiving. It completely wrecked my life.

By the second month of training, I was clocking over twenty miles a week, and I had even run a half marathon by week eight. Seasoned runners eat twenty miles for breakfast before heading out for their leisurely fifty-mile run; I get it—you don't have to remind me. But by the end of the program the only way I could get in enough miles during the week was to ram them all in haphazardly, like taking a load of clothes out of the dryer and just shoving them into drawers without folding them.

Oh, I should probably mention this: I was eating a strict gluten-free vegan diet. Just a minor little detail I left out. Yeah, one of *those* assholes.

How does someone get depressed while eating the cleanest diet on the planet and exercising every day? Spending money to hire a babysitter when you do your long runs on the weekends is a fun way to build resentment, and in my case I was giving up my weekends and paying someone cash so that I could do my least favorite thing in the world. Remind me again why I was doing this: For a good cause? To bring attention to a worthy organization? To brag about it on my deathbed?

Since I live in Utah and we are rarely short on snow during the winter, I did most of my training on a treadmill inside a basement gym at a Jewish community center. I am terrible at running and would otherwise slip on the snow and break my neck. In fact, I did my twenty-mile-long run on a treadmill, and when it was over I thought, *Well that's the most television I have watched in years!*

As much as I can point to deciding to train for this marathon as the beginning of my depression, I can also point to a very specific moment on a beach in Cancún when my outlook on life took a sharp, downward turn. My boyfriend at the time, the second person I dated after my divorce—someone I had started seeing about a month before this depressive episode started—made a series of comments about the amount of food I was eating. Neither of us had our children the week after Christmas in 2015—mine were with my ex and his were with his ex—and we'd traveled to a giant hotel overlooking the Caribbean to try and relax and unplug ourselves from the grind of work and single parenting. But I'd begun my marathon training three weeks prior to this vacation and needed to log nineteen miles in a climate where the humidity was making inanimate objects sweat. One could say that I was hungry, vastly downplaying the mercilessness of my appetite.

My boyfriend didn't have much of an appetite at all, and we were only having one full meal a day. He wasn't really interested in breakfast. Lunch? He'd hesitate and then say he could wait for an early dinner; why couldn't I? I'd packed a few protein bars like I always do but ran out of them by the second day. I was starving, on vacation, in a lovely tropical locale. If I had been an adequately functioning adult in any way, I would have had a conversation with him to communicate the need to fuel my running with food. But I had a very colorful history of suppressing my needs and desires in my relationships with men. It's the reason my marriage ended.

I lived inside a prison that I'd built as a defense mechanism. It's the same prison I'd built in childhood to protect myself from my father's intimidating and unpredictable temper. When I was eight years old,

I once forgot to answer my mother with "Yes, ma'am?" when she called me from across the house. I absentmindedly yelled, "WHAT?" instead—the equivalent of THE HELL DO YOU WANT? in a Southern upbringing—and within seconds my father entered my room, cornered me against a wall, and let his temper roar. His face was mere inches from my own.

"You will not disrespect your mother like that, do you understand me?" he yelled through clenched teeth. "Nod your head and say, 'Yes, sir.'"

The earliest memories I have of my father aren't even of my father. I remember my mother standing in the doorway to their bedroom. She was sobbing and repeating the plea *"Please don't, please don't, please don't"* as my father disciplined my brother. The second memory of my father is of my mother standing in the doorway to the kitchen repeating those same words to him.

In my private sessions with Mel, she had made the correlation and shown me that I was repeating old habits. For years she wanted me to find my voice and defend myself, to own my irreverence, *to simply be me*. To stop being afraid. I feared being cornered against a wall even though my ex hadn't ever intimidated me in any physical way. Although, metaphorically, that was precisely our dynamic. My fierce independence and sometimes brazen personality threatened my ex, and because I always feared that he would shame me for being inappropriate I constantly stifled those parts of myself. He often convinced me that what I was feeling was wrong and bad. I had feared being cornered against a wall in every romantic relationship, but especially with him.

Ironically, training for the first marathon I ever ran back in 2011 signaled the end of my marriage. Hours spent alone on miles of pavement, my bones jolted by every painful step—it all fractured my soul and tore me apart. It exposed all the pain I'd tried to suppress—the pain and stress and exhaustion of remaining vigilant, of making sure I was being appropriate and feeling the *right* things. Less than a month after I crossed the finish line of the 2011 ING New York City Marathon with a broken foot, I asked for a separation. A separation he did not want.

We saw Mel a few times during our separation: he wanted to try to save the relationship, and I wanted help breaking out of it. In our final session we were sitting on a couch opposite her. I was speaking at a tech conference directly after our session and had put on my best clothes and decorated my face with an assortment of makeup I didn't normally wear, details I have to point out because of what happened after she said, "Who wants to start?"

"I'll go," my ex said as he gripped his leg with his very large right hand. "I figured it out," he continued. "I finally figured it out. I have gone over this and over this in my head and now I understand: I am paying for her daddy issues. I am suffering because she hasn't figured out her daddy issues."

He didn't stop there, but I didn't hear the rest of his twenty-minute rant. I had turned my head toward the window to analyze the arthritic curve of a tree branch outside. I thought about winters in Utah, how they expose the bones underneath what was once a blanket of vibrant leaves, brilliant foliage that suddenly surrenders when it's time to go.

When he had stopped talking, Mel turned to me and asked me if I had any response to what he had said. She could see the clenching of my jaw reach all the way to my left temple, and that's when she casually put her hand over her mouth. Maybe that's why I am so drawn to her: because I have no poker face, either. She uses her hand to hide the reaction she must hide as a professional.

And then I let go. I let go of the fear and the worry and the vigilance. I let him know, in no uncertain terms, in a tone that registered on the Richter scale, that my "daddy issues" were the only reason I had remained in our marriage. I had married my father as much as I wanted to believe that I hadn't. And I would be removing myself from this prison cell I had built.

At one point I had to stand up so that the roar in my stomach could make its way out of my throat. Years and years of pent-up resentment echoed throughout the room, going all the way back to the day that he moved in with me—the same day he found out that my ex-boyfriend lived down the hall. He spent *weeks* convincing me that it wasn't normal. Why hadn't I moved? *I should have moved.* Living in an apartment down the hallway from an ex-boyfriend was disrespectful to a current boyfriend, you see. Finally, in that small room overlooking that tree, I yelled, "AND HE WAS PROBABLY GAY! Why did you care?"

Mel was smiling behind her hand. I couldn't see it, but I could see her eyes. I knew that I was giving her what most therapists probably don't ever get to witness in person. I was serving up the fruits of her labor on a platter engraved with the date she'd received her license. I wanted to apologize for the tears and mascara that were dripping onto my nice blouse and the dress pants I'd put on to look like I knew what I was doing when I sat in front of an audience at that tech conference who would hear me speak about writing about life online.

Let the evidence show that I am terrible at communicating my needs in my relationships with men, which is why I am as much to blame for things going wrong as they are, if not more so. Perhaps if I had said to my boyfriend in Cancún that I needed a goddamn sandwich—you know, since I'd run nine miles that morning—I could have curbed the hunger. I could have solved it all with a simple "I am hungry and need to eat." In hindsight it sounds so easy.

Instead I suffered in silence, and when we did eat a meal I would almost resort to using my hands to get the food into my body as fast as possible. I became an obsessed animal, a dumpster raccoon. Over a dinner of beans and rice, he watched as I aggressively scooped every last morsel into my mouth.

"I've never seen anyone eat as much as you do," he said in total disbelief. I set my fork down and tried to swallow my last bite. I felt like someone had punched me in the face, and the force of it caused the room to spin. *I've never seen anyone eat as much as you do.* His words echoed in my ears. And just in case you didn't know this little tidbit about social interaction, let me fill you in on something: Do not ever comment on how or what or when a woman is eating anything. Don't do it. Because you know what might happen? You might trigger an obsession with food that the woman had managed to stifle for over twenty years—an obsession that throttled her ability to function throughout high school and college—all because you couldn't resist monitoring her refried beans. Good job. Well done. Five stars. Ten points for you.

On the final day of our vacation, we chose to read and relax next to the ocean, and when someone from the waitstaff approached us to ask if we'd like anything to eat or drink, my boyfriend's words flashed in giant neon letters at the front of my brain: *I've never seen anyone eat as much as you do.* I calculated the hours before dinner and ordered the largest serving of nachos on the menu so that I could have something to eat throughout the day, to tide me over for nine hours. Yes, the largest serving. The Super Nachos. Los Nachos Más Grandes. He'd already made the rude observation about my appetite, and who was I to prove him wrong?

A half hour later the server returned with a Styrofoam box overflowing with chips and beans and salsa. I had only a few bites, since I was saving most of it to snack on throughout the day and then covered it up with my towel to go for a quick dip with my boyfriend in the ocean. We returned not ten minutes later to a gory crime scene. Chunks of Styrofoam and half-chewed beans littered a twenty-square-foot area. My towel was bunched up in a wadded mass more than four feet from where I had left it. Feathers floated through the air. I quickly pieced together what had happened when two of the culprits showed up again to scrounge for those half-chewed beans.

That's when something snapped in my skull, like a rubber band stretched too far. I ran to my towel, unfolded it so that I could use its full length, and began chasing those seagulls up and down the beach, swinging the towel like a propeller over my head. I am not proud of this. I do not recommend behaving in this manner on a beach where people are trying to unwind. I hope there are no photos or video footage of the crazy white lady in hot pursuit of birds on that one tragic morning in Cancún. But I'm glad I got my energy out, because when I returned to my lounge chair and my boyfriend shook his head and told me through fits of laughter, "You're a little too obsessed with food," I didn't have the energy to cry.

SEVEN
NOTIFICATIONS TO THE NERVOUS SYSTEM

THE DAY AFTER MY second treatment was a Saturday. I woke up to the sound of one of my children rifling through the kitchen drawer where we store the boxes of Honey Nut Cheerios and s'mores-flavor Pop-Tarts that my girls have for breakfast. A week prior to starting treatment, we had moved across town into a house almost 75 percent smaller than the house where I had lived through the entirety of this year-and-a-half-long episode of depression. My bedroom and Marlo's bedroom were located in the basement, and the kitchen was on the ground floor. Now, instead of heading downstairs for breakfast with a directive from the universe to burn it to the ground, she headed *upstairs*, ready to follow through. This also moved us outside the route of Leta's carpool and added to my schedule an hour-long route to drop off both girls at their different schools every weekday. So much Needing to Get Done.

I blinked a few times and could see light shining through the tiny gap between the two panels of blackout shades hanging in my window. I had barely moved during the night. My down comforter lay flat across me as if I'd just tidied my bed. I rolled over to look at the time on my phone and it read 8:24. I couldn't remember the last time I had slept that late, even on weekend mornings when my mother would take my girls to give me a break. My anxiety would wake me up before 7:00 a.m.

More than twenty email notifications cluttered the screen of my phone. Twenty emails overnight. A Friday night. I quickly scrolled through them all, looking for key words like "due" or "denied" or "cannot process" or "invoice." Mostly I was looking for the name of my boss. Whenever I saw the letters of his name on my phone, via either text or email, my entire body would seize. For the previous nine months I had been consulting with a nonprofit working to protect animals. He'd hired me to help overhaul their entire brand and online presence. I brought over twenty years of experience working with Internet-based companies, most notably my blog, which had supported my family for over eleven years. I had pulled back quite a bit from blogging a couple of years previously, given that making money as a blogger had completely transformed. I could no longer make a living off of banner advertisements and instead had to write sponsored content for brands who wanted to insert their products into the stories I was writing about my life and children. I had to manufacture experiences with my kids to fit the talking points of a creative brief and present that as real life.

I knew I just couldn't do it anymore when I was trying to get my kids into the car to play a word game while driving to a ranch in the mountains. This would be the third of three posts I was to write for an automotive brand about quality time with my kids in the car. Except my kids and I don't like to drive long distances or play word games or act even remotely friendly to each other, because *we're confined in a car*. We're either listening to music or staring off in silence or the two of them are bickering about God knows what.

Marlo did not want to participate in yet another ruse, and I had to bribe and threaten and cajole to get her in that car. Right as she opened her door, she looked up at me through tears and begged, "Please, Mom, don't make me do this."

My children had been written into the contract I had with the ad network who negotiated on my behalf with these brands, and I felt dirty and wrong.

When my contract ended with that ad network, I continued to blog a bit, but I turned my focus toward public speaking, an endeavor I thoroughly enjoyed. However, making money as a public speaker is incredibly difficult unless you're a former president or you've discovered the secret to happiness. Not much demand for the opposite of that.

My boss and I had become friends through a mutual friend and connected mostly over our strict vegan diets and concern for animal welfare. When he offered me the job, he knew that I was struggling to book speaking engagements; and when I did speak, the travel completely disrupted my life. I'd booked gigs in Australia, New Zealand, and Germany, and in cities all across the country. Finding child care and someone to watch my dog made arranging travel a nightmare, especially when I had to be somewhere during the school week. It also proved problematic with my marathon training schedule, and on my trip to New Zealand where I spoke at two different conferences, I had to fit in a total of forty training miles. When I returned home, the fatigue of those miles combined with jet lag, and trying to find food that fit my diet left me in a useless heap. Except I didn't really have the option of being a useless heap and instead attempted to tackle All the Things Needing to Get Done like a zombie. Two days later I managed to fit in a sixteen-mile long run on a treadmill.

I accepted the job for the stability of it and signed on as independent contractor so that I could still maintain my own business and pursue any other consulting gigs that might arise. However, it immediately became clear that I would have no time outside of this position to pursue anything, nor would I have the desire to. That's another thing that people don't understand about depression: we don't want to take a shower, we don't know why we feel this way, and even if we did, it wouldn't make us *stop* feeling this way. We have lost all interest in doing anything, especially anything that once brought us joy—because that thing will not bring us joy, and we can't bear the meaning of that. It would be too much. It would crush us.

My boss is one of the most brilliant people I've ever met and had worked in animal welfare for years. He started this nonprofit with a professor in San Diego, and the entire twelve-person team worked remotely. We had employees in California, Oregon, and New York, and three in Salt Lake City. And within that twelve-person team no one really had a firm grasp of the role they were required to play. Meaning: everyone did everything. And often we were working over each other, around each other, and in total darkness. Expectations were nebulous and often miscommunicated or not communicated at all. I'd worked in several Internet start-ups that operated this way—it wasn't a huge surprise to me and I know it's not uncommon elsewhere—except at that time I wasn't raising two daughters by myself. Now I couldn't drop everything to put out a huge fire if I was driving my kid to her piano lesson or picking her up from school because she'd caught yet another cold. Given my circumstances at home, navigating this kind of chaotic work environment proved almost impossible. And my boss would routinely text or email me upset about something that had gone wrong, something that had most likely slipped through the cracks while everyone was trying to figure out what they were supposed to be doing.

After only three months of working with this team, I developed a Pavlovian response to notifications on my phone. Usually these notifications vibrated the watch around my wrist via Bluetooth, and sometimes I would experience what I called ghost vibrations. Even if what I felt was only my shirt sleeve against my arm, I was certain it was a notification, and *what if it was from him?* What had gone wrong? What would I do? How would I fix that problem that I didn't even know existed in the first place? My right hand would shake visibly as I reached for my phone to look at the screen or to tap my watch to see the notification. If I saw his name, I would stop breathing. I feared being cornered against a wall.

I didn't see my boss's name that morning, and swung my legs over the side of the bed to stand up. I hadn't experienced a headache with the second treatment, hadn't hurt or ached since I woke up from the anesthesia the afternoon before. But as I stood up out of the bed, I could feel the bed pulling at my waist, and I sat back down. It was a somewhat familiar feeling, comparable to the fatigue I experienced after a long run in my marathon training. I'd lie down and try to rest, if only just a half hour, but I'd be so anxious that I never fell asleep. And so instead of wasting my time lying there, thinking about All the Things Needing to Get Done, I'd try to get up and start marking things off the list. The exhaustion, however, turned the air around me into peanut butter. I felt somewhat the same that morning, but after greeting my kids in the kitchen I walked over to the couch in the living room and curled up into a ball. A few minutes later I was fast asleep, and for over two hours I had fever dreams of being unable to wake up and fix my kids' lunch, of being unable to wake up and take care of their needs. When I finally forced myself awake, I grabbed my phone off of the coffee table to text my mother.

"I can't really describe it," I mumbled to her when she called me to ask what was wrong. "I feel like the Frankenstein monster. I mean, I feel like I died and someone brought me back to life."

"Heather," she said gently, "you do realize *that's exactly what happened*?"

"Well, yeah, but . . . did I just say that? Except I'm alive and I'm swimming in peanut butter."

I would call this the Peanut Butter Pool, and it happened more than once. It was more than a little discouraging. What if I was always going to feel this way?

EIGHT
LICENSE AND REGISTRATION, PLEASE

THE FOLLOWING DAY MY family gathered at my sister's house for my nephew's farewell. This term is used in the Mormon religion when referring to sending off young men and women on proselytizing missions. He had originally received his "call" to serve in South Africa more than a year before. Sadly, he inherited the all-consuming sadness that afflicts both me and my brother, and he had to defer for a bit because of a severe depressive episode. Somehow my sister escaped the scourge of depression, but it landed smack dab inside the brains of her two siblings. I was the first one in the family to break the silence, to admit that something was wrong and that I needed help. I remember my eleventh-grade AP physics teacher, Ms. Lorraine Jones, stopping class and pulling me into the hallway one afternoon to grab me firmly by the shoulders and warn me, "You can't keep going on like this, Heather. You have to calm down and let go. Otherwise you're going to break." I was first in my class and an all-around horrifying kid to be around. If I didn't ace a test or perform a task perfectly, I thought it meant that I'd end up homeless and alone. This is what my mother called my death spiral: if anything didn't go exactly as planned, I'd end up homeless and alone. And this is another thing to add to the list of things you should know about depression. Depression robs us of the ability to think of anything but the worst possible outcome. Period. It is inevitable. That is the logical end to every thought and action and sequence. What is the point of washing my hair when I'm going to end up sleeping in a cardboard box in a gutter?

Despite her advice, I didn't calm down. Then two months into my sophomore year in college, I broke. I snapped right in half. Yes, I had graduated the valedictorian in high school and was attending college on a full scholarship, but one morning in the fall of 1994 I called my parents to tell them that I was coming home. I was dropping out of college. I could not take it anymore—"it" being breathing air and performing any task that ensured my survival. My depression had eaten me whole, and I was talking to my mother and father from inside its belly. My father, of course, began to tell me to snap out of it. Because I knew that this would be his response, his words starting blurring inside my brain: wah wah wah wah. He'd grown up in the projects of Louisville, Kentucky, only to pull himself up and out of poverty and become a successful manager at IBM, where he would work for over thirty-five years. If he could perform that feat, by God, everyone should be able to. Except I didn't want to breathe air.

My mother, however, had witnessed how depression had wrecked the lives of several of her siblings, and within a week of that phone call she'd made me an appointment with a local psychiatrist. He prescribed me an average dose of Zoloft and within three days my roommates began to tell me that something was different, something was strange. Strange in a *good* way. I hadn't noticed that I was breathing air willingly, and this is one way the medication manifests itself. I didn't realize that I felt better, and when my roommates asked if something had changed, I suddenly thought, *Oh my God!* I'm enjoying this bowl of cereal! The clothes on my body don't hurt! You know, I think I might go outside and smell a flower!

Over a year later I was sitting with my brother, his pregnant wife, and my cousin in a booth at an Olive Garden. We were celebrating my sister-in-law's birthday with unlimited breadsticks, and it didn't take long for my cousin and me to realize that my brother was in one of his moods. Dear Lord, his moods. They would come and go with no warning, pattern, or reason. My brother is the funniest person I know, but he's also the angriest. Angry at what, we never knew. That night he could barely get consonants through his gritted teeth. And when he did, it was only to make mean jokes about my cousin to my cousin's face and then berate the server for bringing a plate of fettuccini when he had *clearly* ordered linguini. After dinner we drove my cousin home, and then I made my brother drop off his wife so that we could speak alone. He drove me to the house I shared with eight roommates and we parked in the driveway.

"What is going on?" I asked after he turned off the engine.

"What do you mean?" he said, clearly surprised that this was the kind of conversation I wanted to have.

"What just happened back there? Did you really need to be that rude? Especially on your wife's birthday? Your *pregnant* wife's birthday?"

He shook his head and mumbled, "I don't know."

"Listen," I said, and turned my entire body to face him, "you're depressed. You have to be. Because if this isn't depression, then you're just the biggest asshole who ever lived."

I hadn't even finished my sentence when he covered his face with both of his hands and starting crying. My big, angry brother. Crying.

"Is that what this is?" he sobbed through his fingers.

"Is this what *what* is?"

He dropped his hands into his lap. "I don't know why I feel this way, Heather. I can't make it stop. Why won't it stop? I don't understand it. I don't want to feel this way, but it just won't stop. I can't control it."

"Ranger," I said, and I reached over to put my hand on his. (Yes, my brother's name is Ranger. He's named after a box of cigars my father saw at a truck stop in Little Rock, Arkansas. Oh, and my sister's name is September even though she was born in January. When I came along they got bored of naming children strangely and picked the name of every other girl born in 1975.) "That's exactly what depression is. You are depressed. *THIS* is depression."

Within a week he saw a psychiatrist, much to the chagrin of my father. It was one thing for his daughter to be "depressed," if that's what I wanted to call it. But it was an entirely other thing for his son to give in to feelings of hopelessness. Not his *son*. Snap out of it, boy. Pull yourself together. If you have no reason to be sad, then you just simply stop being sad. Had he taught us nothing by demonstrating the Herculean feat of his own life?

I still don't think my father acknowledges that the mind is just as susceptible to disease and disorder as any other part of the body: the heart, the lungs, the penis. Even today he doesn't understand that his two children have to struggle with feelings of hopelessness, and that two of my brother's kids, two of my sister's kids, and both of my children suffer from depression and anxiety. My sister had to come up with an alternate explanation as to why her son had deferred his mission, because she couldn't tell my father that he might be suicidal. That would be preposterous. No, actually, not preposterous. Wrong word. That would be *weak*, and his grandson was not weak.

———

My nephew survived that depressive episode, and when he sent in his papers again, the church called him to San Antonio. This thrilled my sister, knowing that if he were to relapse while away from home, he'd at least be in the country and not on the other side of the world. We were gathering at her home to celebrate not only the milestone of his mission but also the fact that, you know, he didn't kill himself. I may not be a practicing Mormon anymore, but I am not a monster (usually) and wanted to show my support for this significant event. I was still swimming in peanut butter as I got dressed that morning and helped Marlo brush her hair, and by the time I got through the controlled chaos of gathering up food for both kids and getting us all into the car, I was exhausted. And *sad*. Profoundly and inexplicably sad.

I wasn't necessarily obsessed with the idea that this wouldn't work—*this* being, of course, willingly dying on a gurney three times a week while my mother watched. But I was worried. That worry hovered in and around me like a noxious gas. Instead of that worry adding to my anxiety, it just made me sad. After I backed out of the driveway and turned out of the tiny secret side street where we'd just moved, I pulled up to a stop sign heading east. Since we'd only been in that neighborhood for a couple of weeks, I was unfamiliar with the traffic traps you learn when you navigate certain roads with frequency. I am also a flagrantly aggressive driver who regards all the rules of the road as merely suggestions. I routinely drive at least

10 miles per hour over the speed limit and can hop a speed bump better than Bo Duke. There are at least three four-way stops on the way to Leta's school in the morning, and because no other human being alive knows how to navigate a four-way stop, my kids know every single four-letter word in the English language.

I pulled up to that stop sign, glanced down at my phone to press PLAY on a music app—DO NOT JUDGE ME; YES, I KNOW BETTER—and slowly rolled through the intersection. Without actually stopping. Zero stopping. I came close, I always do. Right as I looked up from the music app—STOP JUDGING—I caught the silhouette of a cop car to my right. Now, I am a white woman with two young girls in my car. My registration was up-to-date and I had no broken taillights. And yet, the terror that seized me in that moment almost choked the breath out of both of my lungs. My entire face burned bright red with fear and panic and dread, a perfect cocktail of emotion to mix with my sadness. What I so desperately needed to do right then, right as he turned on his lights and siren, was sob.

I pulled over to the side of the road while assuring a now panicked Leta that I was okay, or at least I would be in the future. Not sure if it would be the near future, but eventually. The more I tried to assure her, the harder I cried. The sadness just poured out of me in waves of sobs. By the time the officer approached my window, my entire face was covered in tears and I was shaking. By any measure, I was acting suspiciously. I could be hiding something—anything—and I was either covering it up by pretending sadness or I was genuinely crying because he was just about to discover my wrongdoing. I rolled down the window while simultaneously fumbling through the glove box, looking for my registration, tears splashing the gearshift. I wondered who I would call for bail.

"Hi there," he said, once I had turned my red face toward him. "I'm sure you know that you ran through that intersection back there. I saw you looking at your phone as you ignored the stop sign. And I was right there. You didn't even see me."

Every word of what he was saying was true, except I did see him out of the corner of my eye. Just one millisecond too late. I tried to blink back the tears and was unsuccessful. The only thing I wanted to do as I looked at his face was say, "Please help me. I want to die. I just want to be dead. Please." But Leta would have heard me. Marlo would have heard me. So instead I just bit my lower lip and continued to blink.

"Is everything okay?" he asked, and this is when I thought for sure he was going to ask me to get out of the car so that he could search it. He wouldn't find any drugs or severed heads, but he would find a shit ton of used tissues. He'd find dirty socks, two umbrellas that didn't open, months of old graded homework tucked into the spaces between each seat, and several hundred gas receipts I will one day file in a folder labeled "Gas Receipts."

"I just . . ." I didn't know how to answer him. Anything other than telling him that this whole giant mess sitting in front of him was just a simple case of wanting to be dead would be a total lie. "I have had . . ."

He could tell that I was having a hard time getting words out my mouth. "Have you had a bad day?"

I involuntarily and immediately nodded my head and choked in a sob.

"Let me have your license and registration and I'll be right back, okay? Just sit tight." He then patted his hand on the door, a reassuring gesture, as if everything would be all right.

The three of us sat in silence while he retreated to his car. I reached over and grabbed Leta's hand to try to comfort her, if that was even possible, given my emotional state and the fact that law enforcement was now involved.

In my side mirror I saw him get back out of his car to approach me again. My heart began racing and I could feel the rhythm of it in my neck against the collar on my shirt. When he got to my door, he patted it again before speaking.

"Listen, I'm going to let you go and urge you to heed that stop sign next time, okay?" He handed me my license and registration. "I hope your day gets better," he continued, and then he pointed first to Leta and then to Marlo in the back seat. "Are these your girls?"

I glanced around at both of them and then faced him. "Yes. Yes, they are."

"Beautiful children," he said. "You all have a good day." He patted the door one last time and then he left. He turned and walked back to his car. I marveled at the nature of that entire interaction, starting with the fact that my panic and fear arose only from the idea of getting a ticket or, at worst, having my car searched. I did not once fear for my life (despite wanting to be dead) or the lives of my children. And then *he showed me compassion*. He offered me comfort. He patted my goddamn door three separate times. I got to drive away from that encounter without a ticket, and he wished me well. If only every person's traffic stop were so earnestly rosy and not, you know, fraught with the idea that they might have their face blown off.

When I arrived at my sister's house a half hour later, the kids ran in before me. My face was swollen from all of that stupid, hysterical crying, and when I walked in the door I immediately went into a sitting room to the left of the entryway. I set my purse down next to a desk and then plopped myself on the floor beside it. A cacophony of voices filled the house: siblings, cousins, aunts and uncles, grandchildren, my father and stepmother. I knew everyone was feasting on a buffet of potluck dishes, despite no sounds of cutlery hitting plates. Hillbilly to the core, we use plastic knives and forks, paper plates, and red Solo cups. Everyone would take home leftovers wrapped in tinfoil.

Suddenly my mother rounded the corner. "There you are," she said as she finished chewing a piece of food. She was wiping her hands with a paper towel. "I saw Leta and Marlo come in; they said you were right behind them." Seeing her face and hearing her voice instigated that thing that happens between a mother and her children, that safe feeling wherein all the pent-up emotion from a horrible day at school—all the emotion you've hidden from classmates and teachers and coaches—all comes suddenly rushing to the surface.

I pulled my legs in to my chest and rested my head on my knees to cry. "I got pulled over for running a stop sign," I wept, with a bit of a laugh thrown in. I then lifted my head to look at her. "And it's fine, you know, he was perfectly lovely. He didn't even give me a ticket and complimented the kids, but look at me! I'm a mess!"

She walked over to me to rest her hand on my head. "Heather, anyone would be—"

"But I'm still like this! I mean, I've gone under twice now, and for what? What am I doing? Why am I risking this if it isn't going to work?"

"You're only two treatments in, honey. We have to give this—"

"Give this *what*? I'm stealing hours of your life away from you to do this, and I still can't handle anything. I can't get over the hurdle. *I still can't handle anything.* This isn't fair to you!"

"Remember what I told you," she said, and then reached down to cradle my chin in her hand. "We are doing this. We are doing whatever it takes. *Whatever it takes.* Two treatments down, eight to go. We have nothing else to do this month other than be there when you wake up. Do you hear me?"

I nodded and then the hillbilly took over and I wiped my face on the sleeve of my jacket. "I just don't want to feel like this anymore. That's it. That's all I want." I just wanted to be able to handle things. To be free of the malaise I felt at the idea of tackling anything. *Anything*. It could be something as insignificant as ironing a shirt or unloading the dishwasher. Sometimes the idea of having to lace up a pair of boots was too much. And it wasn't just the effort of it, although that was a large part of it. It was also the *why* of it. Why lace up these boots when I didn't want to leave the house in the first place? Why iron this shirt when I didn't want to get dressed? If no one else could smell the coffee-stained T-shirt I'd been wearing for three days in a row, what was the problem?

But the significant things—remaining calm when your seven-year-old is banging her head on the keys of the piano, a plumbing problem arises with the kitchen sink, a deadline looms, you're getting pulled over for running a stop sign—these things might as well be at the top of a 120-story building when the elevator is broken. And so are your legs. Depression extinguishes our purpose in life—the purpose of *anything* in our lives—making it quite literally impossible to handle anything. Every day and hour and minute is an obstacle course of things we are supposed to handle; most people do so without any effort, but we can't even see around the first corner. And so we collapse. Or we sleep for days on end. Or we yell at people who don't deserve it. Some of us drink ourselves into a stupor. Others scream into a pillow or crawl into a corner to rock back and forth. Some of us retreat to a closet to call their mother and say, "Please, let me be dead."

NINE

THE LIE OF A SUICIDAL IDEATION

THE FOLLOWING MORNING I drove my kids to school on an empty stomach. The clinic had called to let me know that I'd need to come in for the third treatment that afternoon at 1:00 p.m. I would have my final glass of water before leaving the house, before approaching that stop sign and bringing the car to a full stop for ten seconds.

"Mom, you can go. There are no cars coming," Leta said, looking at me like only a seventh grader can.

"Yes, I am aware," I shot back. "But if you will recall, yesterday we had a little run-in with law enforcement, and I'd rather not repeat that."

I pulled out into the intersection and continued on the route we took to her school every morning. A few minutes passed before she asked, "So, are Grandmommy and Grandpa Rob coming over today? I mean, to help you?"

She knew more than Marlo knew, but she didn't know any of the details. She knew that my mother and stepfather were taking me to a clinic every other day "to help with my anxiety," and she knew that they stayed after they brought me home so that I could take a short nap. She did not know that they both watched me fall swiftly under the grip of propofol anesthesia into the abyss where I would remain for over fifteen minutes. She didn't know about the needle, the breathing tube, the Zofran, or the lidocaine. She didn't know about the recovery room or the crazy shit that would come out of my mouth in the drunken minutes after I awoke. She didn't know about Greg or Chris or Molly or Dr. Tadler or Dr. Mickey. She didn't know about the wire affixed to my forehead with Velcro. She didn't need to know these things, and not just because she might slip and say something to her father. She just needed to know that I wanted to get better and that I was trying to get better, because the one thing she did know was that I was unhappy. Although she did not know the extent of my unhappiness, she could see the hopelessness etched into every line of my face.

When I pulled up along the curb where parents drop off their seventh- and eighth-grade kids, she strapped her backpack to her right shoulder and then dramatically turned to face me.

"Good luck today," she said.

"Thank you, honey," I said, and reached over to pull her into an embrace over the center console of the car. "Everything will be fine."

I repeated that line again and again—"Everything will be fine . . . Everything will be fine . . . Everything will be fine"—after filling out the questionnaire and receiving my identity bracelet from Greg. My answers were the same as they had been when I filled it out the previous Friday, and I lingered probably a little too long on number 5, the bullet point assessing my level of sadness. That word is not one I had ever used to describe my mental health in the previous year. "Hopeless," "anxious," "irritable," "angry," "panicked," "depressed"—

all of these dominated my vocabulary when I talked to my mother or my therapist. But up until I'd seen that specific question the first time, I don't think I had linked the word "sad" to what I had been experiencing. Yet it so perfectly summarized how I felt about being alive: I was sad.

My mother was talking to me about a few of our family members and the conversations she'd had with them the previous day at the farewell party, and I was mostly paying attention. Spending this much time with her made me realize that as she has gotten older her manic energy expresses itself less in a constant need to move and more through a constant need to talk. She talked endlessly, breathlessly, sometimes weaving her way through three stories at once. Often I would look over at my stepfather during these rambling narratives to see him gleefully staring off into the distance because he'd been relieved for once of having to be her audience.

She was saying something about my nephew, but I got distracted by a few of the ECT patients sitting in the waiting room with us. Some of them were acting and talking like the stereotypes we imagine when we think of electroconvulsive therapy. Some were clearly disoriented; one looked like he hadn't slept in months. One woman's hands were trembling so badly that she could barely hold the pen to fill out her paperwork. I probably looked exactly like all three of them rolled into one.

We shared the waiting room with the final ECT patients of the day. On one occasion I would come in for my treatment after the clinic had completed twenty-two ECT appointments. They have that procedure down to a minute-by-minute precision and know how long it will take each person to complete a round. My treatment, however, was a little less polished, and understandably so. I was only the third person to qualify for and agree to participate in the study.

I would not know for several weeks that every technician and nurse and doctor and anesthesiologist helping me was donating their time. They stayed a few hours after the last ECT appointment *without extra compensation*. The ultimate goal of this study, Dr. Mickey explained to my mother when I was under anesthesia for my second treatment, was to provide proof that an anesthetic can offer the benefits of ECT without the side effects of ECT. The most debilitating of these are short-term or permanent memory loss and migraines. Because my psychiatrist had assembled an incredible team, none of them hesitated when asked if they'd volunteer to help Dr. Mickey.

We waited for over an hour that day due to some delays with the ECT patients going before me, and my stomach grumbled so loudly, it sounded like a scene in a cartoon. It almost drowned out my mother's talking—conversation that, let's be honest, I didn't mind at all. It was a distraction from everything: the hunger and the thirst, the needle, the drugs and the tubes and the vials, the sadness, and the worry that all of this might be a huge waste of everyone's time.

When she reached a natural pause in her monologue, I asked, "I don't want to change the subject, but can you help me make sure to remind them about the fentanyl?"

"Of course," she said. "I'm sure they have it written down some-where, but I'll say something."

"And . . . can you help me talk to them about . . . it's been six days now. Six days. This isn't normal."

"Six days . . . since?" She was confused.

"Six days since I last . . . you know . . ." I opened my eyes as wide as I could and wobbled my head around. I really hate talking about my bathroom habits with anyone, even my mother. I spent so many years of my life invested in the pattern and consistency of my chil-dren's bowel movements and have written tomes about the subject on my website. And because of that I don't ever want to waste another minute discussing the topic.

"Hm . . ." My mother pursed her lips. "It could be that you're having to go so long without eating anything. You're having to skip one or two meals every other day."

"Yeah," I said. "But I am still eating food. And I haven't felt a single urge in six days. I just don't feel normal that way."

"Let's ask Dr. Mickey if anything they're giving you might be causing this." I was so glad to have her there, to have her voice—however talkative—and her advocacy. She made me feel safe. The few friends I'd told about the treatment knew that I'd taken a huge leap of faith in agreeing to do it, and whenever any of them uttered a "Whoa . . ." I'd say, "My mom will be there. I'll be okay."

When they finally called me in for prep, I didn't recognize the phlebotomist. I was starving and my tongue kept getting stuck to the roof of my mouth from the dehydration. I took my seat across the room from a giant television. The first time I sat in that room a loop of landscapes in Hawaii played. I recognized a specific beach I'd visited in Maui, a girls' trip I'd taken three years before to support my friend whose fiancé had committed suicide just days after proposing. The day it happened, my stylist was finishing up my routine haircut when I got the phone call from a mutual friend. They'd found his body in the trunk of his car. It was parked at a train station. He had climbed inside it and taken his life. Those were the straightforward details, but the why of it all was so confusing to her. To everyone. That night I bought enough Thai food to feed the group of friends who would gather at her house to comfort and talk and *just be there for her*. When I walked in she got up from her seat, walked over to me, and collapsed into my arms. I held her for several minutes and stroked her hair. She then pulled me by my right arm to take me to her bedroom, where we could talk alone. She knew and I knew that I was perhaps the only one there who could give her some insight into the why of it all. She knew I'd once been that desperate.

She talked about the conflict he'd been feeling about leaving the religion he'd known and practiced his entire life. She talked about the conflict he'd been feeling about extracting himself from a loveless marriage and his constant worry over what that might do to his three kids. She talked about his depression, how he seemed to be managing it. How could he do this to her? How could he do this to his three kids? How? Why? *How could he do this to them?*

I let her talk and wail and sob. Her eyes were almost swollen shut from the crying. And then I held her hands and said, "I know you and everyone else think that he did this, this *something*, to you, to his kids. But I will tell you right now that in order for him to make the decision to get into that trunk and do what he did, he had to have been deceived. The depression had deluded him into thinking that all of you would be better off without him. The depression convinced him of that. The depression made him believe that he was relieving all of you from the burden of himself. The depression did this. *He* did not do this."

Some friends tried to console her with the notion that he'd been selfish, that he'd betrayed her and the love they had for each other. Months later she would tell me that what I had offered her that night in her room was one of the things that had given her a glimmer of peace. And yet, there I sat, waiting to have a 22-gauge needle inserted into my arm, watching images of rain forests and flowers loop on the enormous TV across the room, thoroughly convinced that everyone in my life would be better off without me. It was a truth my addled brain could not refute.

This was the friend I had called one night two months prior to starting treatment when I found myself in my bathtub wondering if I could will myself to remain underneath the water. My phone was on the floor next to the tub and with wet fingers I texted, "I think you should probably come over here. I shouldn't be alone." And then I felt terrible for having put that pressure on her and fired off another text immediately. "Actually, I'm fine. Don't come over."

My phone starting ringing before I set it back on the floor, and when I saw her name I hesitated only briefly.

"Hey," I answered.

"I am coming over right now, goddamnit," she howled into her phone. "And you better open that fucking door." She knew she could use that language with me, and she was using it half jokingly, half "Do not make me call the cops on you." Ten minutes later after I'd toweled off and slipped on a T-shirt and yoga pants that I found on the floor next to my bed, I let her in and grabbed her. She nodded in my neck as I cried, and then she led me back to my bed. I climbed in first and then she climbed in behind me and whispered as she stroked my hair, "I'm staying all night. I'll be here all night." Early the following morning she got up, mentioned a meeting she had to get to, and told me how much she loved me. I am so glad I opened that door.

I didn't really have the desire to get to know this third phlebotomist, and she wasn't trying to interact with me as I sat staring at the screen. She was older than Molly, with shoulder-length hair, and she wore a stiff white coat. As she prepared all the materials, the mood in the room felt sterile and cold. She ran through the list of my medications rather quickly, and I didn't tell her about my urinary tract and its unique shape. I didn't tell her that wanting to be dead destroys one's sex drive and that I couldn't remember what it felt like to want to be intimate with someone. That the thought of having to wash my hair was reason enough not to go on a date.

And then she stood up from her seat at the computer, snapped on a pair of rubber gloves, and picked up the needle. I showed her the yellowing bruises on my right arm from the previous two treatments and asked if she could try my left arm. She walked around to the other side of my body, affixed a rubber tourniquet to my upper arm, and asked me to make a fist. I flexed my hand several times and my super-veins bulged like giant blue pipes underneath my skin. I turned my head when I saw her make a movement toward my arm, and then my entire body seized with the jab of it, like she'd hacked into my arm with a saw. I tried not to groan, but then she jabbed at a vein again, and again I could feel the pain shoot up into the back of my jaw. I took several quick, sharp breaths and closed my eyes. She apologized, said she couldn't get the needle all the way in and would need to try it one more time. I clenched my right hand around my thigh to brace for it, but nothing could have prepared me for that third attempt. I involuntarily let out a moan and tried to hide it with my breath. My entire left arm was on fire.

"I don't know what's wrong," she mused. "I can get the needle into the vein; I just can't get it as far in as it's supposed to be. Let me go find my colleague." She swiftly exited the room, and I immediately threw back my head and groaned at the ceiling. This loosened the grip between the roof of my mouth and my tongue, and I thought about how amazing a swig of apple juice would feel in my throat. After a few minutes she returned with another woman in a white coat, someone I'd seen before walking through the halls of the clinic.

She picked up my left arm and examined my veins, turning my arm from left to right.

"Have you tried the other arm?" she asked

"You used my right arm the last two times!" I interjected, panicky from the thought of having the needle aimed at my bruises. I picked up my arm to show her the injection sites.

She inspected the wounds on my right arm and let out a heavy sigh. "Okay, let's try this arm one more time. Here," she said, turning to the original phlebotomist, "hold her arm like this and I'll try this vein." She pointed to one that had grown purple and now resembled an earthworm. The original phlebotomist held my arm out straight and gripped it so that I couldn't move it. I turned my head and felt the saw in my arm. She struggled with it a bit and the entire left side of my head buzzed in pain. After a few more seconds of wriggling the needle into place, she placed both of her hands on her hips and said, "With *your* veins, you'd think we wouldn't even need to be trained to do this. Sorry about that! This needle is not a fun one."

Ha! Haha! Not a fun one! This needle was becoming the worst part of the entire death experience.

I returned to the waiting room with purple paper tape wrapped around my left arm and slouched into the seat next to my mother. Just then a nurse walked in and asked if I was ready. This is when I wished that time would slow down, because the time between walking out of the waiting room to the time that the propofol would overcome me felt like a scene being fast-forwarded. I wanted to take in all the details of the experience, but a treatment this serious doesn't fuss around with nonsense.

The nurse led me to the gurney while asking my name and birthday. I always had to resist answering, "Don't you know who I am?" Because that joke doesn't ever get old. Even Leta makes this joke about me. If we get bad service at a fast-food restaurant, she'll whisper to me, "Don't they know who you are? TELL THEM WHO YOU ARE." And I'm, like, "Leta. 'I am the Mommy Blogger' isn't going to get us your chicken nuggets any faster."

I told the room my name and hopped up on the gurney, and then I asked for the warm blanket, since they had forgotten to offer it. The team began affixing all the various instruments to my body, a precise series of maneuvers involving Velcro and vials and tubes and tiny adjustments. I looked at my mother, who was standing next to Dr. Mickey, and blinked several times to remind her about the constipation. They were ready to start the treatment—it had not even been two minutes since I was sitting in the waiting room—when my mother put her hand on Dr. Mickey's arm.

"Hey, guys," she began. "It's time to talk about poop."

"Oh my God," I said, the Velcro from the wire itching my forehead. "Are you seriously—"

"Oh, so NOW you're a prude? I don't think so," she shot back. "Yes, today we are gonna talk about poop. Specifically, Heather's poop. Could there be anything in the combination of drugs you're giving her that could cause constipation? She hasn't pooped since she started the study."

"Mom, how many years have you been waiting to do this to me?"

"I would have done this at your wedding, but you eloped."

I could see Dr. Mickey going through the list of drugs in his brain and on his fingers. This one? No. That one? No. He turned to the anesthesiologist on call that day, Dr. Beck, who furrowed his brow.

"Well, you are having to go long periods without eating food," Dr. Beck said. "But we can do some research before you come in next time to see if we can find anything."

"In the meantime," my mother said as she walked over to place her hand on my foot, "I have some poop tea I can give her. We'll fix you some poop tea today, okay?" And then she winked at me.

And with that final pronouncement about the poop tea, it was time to die.

Dr. Beck asked me if I was ready for the Zofran and lidocaine. I nodded and clenched my hands against my chest. My mother was still standing at the foot of my gurney, her hands now behind her back. I sought out her eyes and she found mine.

"And here's the propofol," he said as he held up the milky liquid. I glanced quickly at the vial, and then found my mother's face again. Out of the corner of my eye I could see him exerting pressure on the vial. *How long could I withstand it?* I wondered again. *Could I will myself to stay awake?* Several seconds passed and I didn't feel anything, so I looked around the room to see if everyone could see that I was willing myself to stay aw—

Nothingness.

Then suddenly I could feel the weight of someone's hand on my left leg. I could feel that I was not lying flat, that my body was propped up. I blinked a few times and found it very difficult to swallow. My mouth was parched. I didn't recognize the person sitting to my right and blurted, "Who are you? What are you doing here? Why are you going around scaring people like this?"

That drunk girl at the party.

"You don't remember me? We met last time. I'm Chris," he said. His voice was so gentle that I suddenly felt like a jerk.

"Wait . . . Chris? Chris. Chrissssssss. *Chrisopher.* Yeah. Heeeeyyy!"

He smiled. "Can you tell me your name?"

"Heather Armstrong. Wait, Heather *B.* Armstrong."

"Great. Can you tell me what year it is?"

"Two thousand and twelve."

"Hm . . . can you think about that a little more?" he asked.

"One, two, three . . ." I looked down at my fingers to count. "It's 2012." Everyone in the room got silent again, all of them exchanging glances. "Oh, for fuck's sake. Did I get it wrong again?"

"Try one more time," my mother said. I saw that it was her hand on my leg.

I closed my eyes and could see clock gears shifting around, interlocking with each other until the number "2017" suddenly appeared in my head.

"Oh my God, I am so embarrassed. It's 2017. Sorry."

"Don't apologize," Chris offered. "This happens a lot. We just want to make sure you're fully awake before we let you go anywhere."

"Where's my damn apple juice?" I said jokingly, slamming my fist on my thigh. Another nurse took a container out of a small refrigerator at the other side of the room and poured some into a plastic cup. "I'm going to need more than that!" I hollered.

My mother, who hasn't ever really witnessed me when I'm drunk, said, "Heather, she can pour you another cup after you've finished this one."

"I KNOW THAT, MOTHER," I said. "But I can't control what comes out of my mouth—oh God. Poop tea! You talked about my poop in front of everyone. Why do I have to remember this? Here I am all '2012,' but I can't forget poop tea?"

She was cackling at this point, because I was bringing China Slim Tea, Extra Strength, Herbal Tea Delight up in front of two recovery nurses who had not been privy to the original conversation. "Heather is constipated," she said to Chris.

"MOM—"

"And we're trying to figure out if it's a side effect of one of the drugs. Heather, there is an Asian market around the corner from your house. We'll stop there on the way home to pick up your poop tea."

After two more cups of apple juice that I drank without taking a breath, I swung my legs over the gurney and stood up. My stepfather steadied me, and he and I walked arm in arm out into the long hallway, out into the parking lot. I could hear my mother lingering behind, telling one of the nurses to remind Dr. Mickey about checking into the medications. She caught up with us just as my stepfather was about to open that giant minivan door and I caught a glimpse of my face in the window. I reached out to touch it. In the haze of drunken, incorrect years and poop talk I suddenly realized: Wait. *Wait.* I'd taken two showers in the last four days. Two. And put on makeup. How I hadn't realized the significance of this as I was doing it, I cannot know. I reached my hand out to touch the reflection of my face where I'd applied mascara that morning and traced the two gaping holes where my eyes used to be.

TEN

A BOWL OF CHIPS AND SALSA

WE DIDN'T GET HOME until almost 4:30 that afternoon. I had not eaten food since 8:00 the previous night, so I'd essentially been fasting for twenty straight hours. I gobbled a 20-gram protein bar in the car on the drive to my house—I made actual "gobble" sounds, like a turkey—and when I walked in the door, Marlo was sitting at the countertop next to her babysitter, Lyndsey. Friends who knew about the treatment asked how I was going to manage my girls during these weeks, and the truth is that all of us just agreed that we'd wing it. When I say "all of us," that includes Lyndsey. I had hired her at the beginning of the school year to pick up my girls from school, bring them home, and stay with them until 5:30 every night so that I could get in a full day of work. She helped Marlo with her homework, prepared snacks for both kids, and kept them entertained so that I didn't lose my mind trying to manage all of that with my workload and a boss who randomly texted that a certain form on the website was broken and why had I not fixed it already? A form so buried inside a maze of menus that no one in the world had ever used it or even seen it except for me and him.

Lyndsey is the last in a long line of babysitters who have helped me out over the years. First there was Katey, and then my niece Mariah. There was my adopted sister Cami who used to drive up from Provo, Utah, on the weekends to help out with Marlo. My cousin McKenzie lived with us for almost a year, and unfortunately Marlo came to believe that McKenzie was hers and hers alone. She believed that she was owed an *actual person*. When Kenzie got married and then pregnant, she couldn't care for Marlo anymore, and I hired a girl named Kelli to pick the girls up from school and help with homework. And then Marlo thought Kelli was now Her Person. Hers alone. Whenever I tried having a conversation with Kelli in the afternoons, Marlo would talk over us or, you know, scream and kick walls. Sometimes she screeched and threw her body on the floor. I'm a pretty strict parent, stricter than a lot of my friends, and I don't normally let my children get away with this kind of behavior. But when her father moved across the country, I eased up on a few things. In the case of Marlo owning Kelli, I figured that I didn't need to further distress the edges of that enormous vacancy. I quickly learned that the best way to have a conversation with Kelli was to text her to meet me in the bathroom. There we would whisper or flush the toilet to mask the sounds of our voices.

When Kelli left to do corporate work, I found Lyndsey. After the second treatment I let her know exactly where I was going to be three days a week. Flatlining! On the Michael Jackson drug! Obstinately saying crazy nonsense to strange nurses! Her reaction was similar to those I'd already confided in: a little dubious, but "Do what you gotta do." She didn't know the Wanting to Be

Dead part, but she could tell that I'd seemed a bit down. Haha! Ha. Yes. Down.

When I walked in that afternoon, the combination of hunger and fatigue must have made me look somewhat strange. I came to this conclusion when Lyndsey startled so visibly that the stool she sat on scooted two inches. She asked if I was okay, and I nodded and pointed toward the basement, where I really wanted to be. Right then, in my bed: Just let me be in my bed. I walked over to Marlo, kissed her on the forehead, and somehow found the strength to turn to my mother, who had walked in behind me, to say, "Please tell Leta I love her. I have to go lie down."

I stumbled down the stairs into my bedroom and crawled underneath the covers, but not before setting my alarm for 5:30 p.m. I was too tired to eat anything, even though my roaring stomach was barely muffled through my duvet. An hour would be plenty; I just had to close my eyes. Dr. Bushnell sold me on this clinical trial by telling me it would work. But he also promised that I'd finish up each treatment and be able to go about my normal life, and this fatigue kept happening. All three times I'd been so tired on the car ride home that my head would bob with each turn and stop. And there in my bed I instantly fell asleep, my phone still aglow in my hand.

When my alarm went off, I didn't know where I was. My room was almost pitch-black, save for a tiny space in the curtains letting in the diminishing light outside. I had to blink several times to get my bearings, and then I heard the scuffling of feet upstairs and the muffled voice of my mother saying goodbye to Lyndsey. My village was tag-teaming.

I pulled the heaviness of my body up and out of the bed—the Peanut Butter Pool—and climbed the stairs into the blinding light of the kitchen. My mother was wiping up something on the counter, when she turned to me and saw me covering my eyes with my hand.

"Why don't you go back to sleep? We've got everything covered," she said.

Asking for help still didn't feel right or normal. In fact, it still felt downright weak, and I hated that I was consuming so much of her life. "I'm okay," I said. "I want to see the kids. Where are the girls?"

Both of them had finished up their homework and were snuggled up together on Leta's bed. Leta was on her phone, Marlo on an iPad I'd bought for her on sale at Christmas. The two of them, always seeking each other out in quiet moments. Always hugging and sharing things they'd discovered, always ending up on the couch or the bed, a leg or an arm entwined. Marlo was born early on a Sunday morning, and I remember the following Saturday being overcome by a feeling of sorrow and regret. I truly believed that I had ruined Leta's life by burdening her with a little sister—a sibling she might or might not like, a younger human she'd be stuck with for the rest of her life. Why had I done this to her? What had I been thinking the whole nine months I'd carried that strange, wriggling eventuality in my womb? Why had I not given my five-year-old a say in whether or not she should have to be related to a sister? It was all my fault: she would end up homeless and alone. Coincidentally, the following Monday I started taking a load of antidepressants again.

I sat down at the foot of Leta's bed as she put down her phone to hug me. I felt bad that I had been too tired to find her when I'd gotten home. Our afternoon ritual included a hug the moment she walked in from school. Always a long, lingering hug. Didn't matter if I was on a conference call or in the middle of calculating quarterly taxes: I would stop whatever I was doing as she'd run in to hug me. Marlo? She had Her Person, and that person was giving her undivided attention. She would get to me later when she needed more undivided attention, plus ice cream.

"How did it go?" Leta asked, and her voice wavered a bit. I hated that my firstborn child was as worried as I was that I might not ever again smile the way I used to.

"Good," I assured her. "Everything is good." I pulled her in tightly and stroked the back of her head just as my mother rounded the corner and poked her head through the doorway.

"Rob and I are going to get them a pizza and then we're going to stay and help put Marlo to bed," she announced. "You have no say in this, so don't open your mouth. Also, I've put a load of laundry in and it'll be done and put away before we leave." She then held up her hand as if to stop traffic.

––––––––––––

My mother had always been my backup since my divorce, especially since my ex had moved and I started doing all of this alone. But it wasn't until I asked my mother to come to a therapy session with me about three months before the treatment that she finally understood the extent of what doing all of this alone had done to me. I didn't want her to come to a session. It meant I'd be asking for help, and I couldn't do that. I didn't want to admit that I desperately needed the occasional extra set of hands. My therapist, Mel, said that if I didn't have her come in, she would track my mother down and call her in herself. Illegal? Probably. But it was a good tactic, and Mel knew it would be.

So I called my mother and asked if she would accompany me

to one of my weekly sessions. She didn't hesitate, given, you know, all the phone calls and screaming and the once or twice I might have mentioned that I wanted to be dead. On a snowy Wednesday afternoon in December we pulled into the parking garage of my therapist's building.

"We can take the elevator if you want," I said as we approached the entrance. "But I usually take the stairs, and those five flights are no joke."

"Is that a challenge?" my mother shot back. "I may be old, but I am not *old*. Do I need to remind you how many times you've ever beaten me in steps? And that the only two times were, first, when you cheated and, second, when I was undergoing radiation for my breast cancer?"

"Stairs it is!" I enthusiastically cheered, to distract my brain from the memory of my ex claiming that my mother's "newly diagnosed medical condition" would render her incapable of helping me take care of my children. It was yet another reason he thought I was unfit to be their mother. Little did he know that during the four months that my mother endured radiation, she clocked more than 15,000 steps each and every day.

We entered the cold concrete corridor of stairs and slowly ascended to the fifth floor. These stairs, like I said, were no joke. In fact, when my therapist had moved her office a few months earlier, I realized that each floor was so high above the one below it that every set of stairs equaled two flights. Counting the stairs that went down into the parking garage, the five-story building offered approximately twelve flights of stairs.

Three times a week I'd walk Marlo to the door of her classroom and then drive five blocks down the street to this office building, where I would trespass those twelve flights of stairs twelve times, my iPhone strapped to my waist with a workout band I'd bought while training for the Boston Marathon. I'd listen to a running playlist of more than two hundred embarrassingly awful pop songs and fly up and down those stairs, always making sure to avoid eye contact with anyone entering the stairwell heading to their professional office. This would make them believe that a woman dressed entirely in workout clothing and white earbuds with sweat pouring from her temples belonged in that stairwell more than anyone had ever belonged, so please don't call the cops.

My therapist's office sat at the end of a long hallway on the fifth floor, and my mother and I walked toward it in silence. Neither one of us knew quite what to expect. I'd freshened up a tiny bit by wearing a pair of yoga pants that could pass as gray slacks and put on an old sweater I used to wear when I hated myself less. My mother, as always, was dressed as if she would be briefing the president about an air strike. (She doesn't walk to her mailbox without ironing her shirt and putting on lipstick.) When we reached Mel's office, we sat in the waiting room in silence. I think I may have fibbed a little earlier, because I knew a bit of what to expect. Remember: me, china shop. Mel, bull.

Fifteen minutes later—because of course we'd arrived fifteen minutes early—Mel opened the door to her office to let a couple—a tall, dark-haired man and a much shorter woman with a blond bob—exit. Mel's specialty is marriage counseling, but she'd kept me as a client after my divorce because she knew the ins and outs of my brain so well. I tried not to make eye contact with the couple. I thought, *Are they going to see me and my mother sitting here and think,* That is the strangest pair of lesbians I have ever laid eyes on?

They passed us as Mel approached, a giant smile on her face. I caught the glimmer in her eye, like, *My, my, my. So this is Heather's mom. Of course she is.*

"You must be Linda," she said, beaming, reaching out to shake my mother's hand. My mother stood up and grabbed Mel's hand first with her right hand and then placed her left hand on top to emphasize what this moment meant to her. There was going to be so much crying in that room, I just knew it. Stop it with the warm, meaningful embraces, ladies, while I'm wanting to be dead.

"Yes," my mother answered. "Thank you so much for having me, and *thank you so much* for what you've done for Heather."

Mel flashed a bewildered glance at me and said, "Well, of course! That's what she pays me to do!"

We followed her into her office overlooking the eastern half of the valley, the Wasatch Front stretching from north to south. I took my usual seat on the far side of the sectional next to the orange blanket with tassels. My mother sat down on the other side of the sectional, set down her purse, and then straightened out her shirt and the dress coat she was wearing over it. Mel took her seat across from us both, leaned back, and crossed her legs. After an audible exhale, she looked straight at me and asked, "Does she know why she's here?"

I shrugged and mumbled, "She knows a little bit—"

"I know she's been seeing you every week for the last several months," my mother interjected. "I know we need to do something—"

"Your daughter needs help. She needs *your* help. I asked her to bring you here because she is too afraid to ask you. So I am going to make her ask you."

"She knows I would do anything—" My mother had negotiated with CEOs and the presidents of international corporations, but she'd never met Mel.

"Yes, she knows all of that." Mel waved her hand around. "But she can't say the words or reach out when she needs to reach out. For a list of reasons. Do you know how bad this has gotten?"

"She has told me how she feels, yes. Things are not good."

"Right. But do you know how bad this has gotten?"

"Things are really bad . . ."

"If we don't figure out a plan today, right now, your daughter is going to end up in a hospital if she even makes it there alive. And my goal—*our* goal—is to figure out a way for her to handle the impossible, the unfathomable, load that she carries so that her ex doesn't come along and claim that she is an inadequate mother. We don't want her to lose her life." She smiled in my direction. "But, more importantly, we will not let her lose her children."

My mother began to tear up. "Heather and I have talked about this. She's scared he's going to find out that she's depressed. I know she is more scared of that than anything else."

"Frankly, that's the thing I, too, am most scared about for her. She's stuck in a catch-22: if she seeks any sort of major treatment, he's going to find out. But she can't get better if she doesn't get some help."

"We've talked about this, too, yes."

"That's where you come in."

"I want to help her, but I don't know what to do! Tell me what to do! I can't diagnose her—"

"Heather," Mel interrupted. "Tell her. Tell her what you need most."

I blinked back my tears and fiddled with the tassels on the blanket. I bit my lower lip as I swallowed a giant sob. "I've told her that I'm drowning in the day-to-day of things."

"Yes, but get specific."

I leaned forward and stuck my elbows on my legs so that I could hide my face with my hands. "I cannot comprehend how I am going to unload the dishwasher one more time, Mom. I cannot comprehend how I am going to do one more load of laundry. I cannot comprehend how I am going to help Marlo practice one more song. I cannot comprehend the logistics of taking a shower. I cannot comprehend how I am going to get up tomorrow and do it again and again and again." I removed my hands from my face so that I could gesture to indicate the magnitude of what I was about to say. "This hamster wheel I'm on, I can't escape it for even a second." I spread my arms as wide as they would go, and then leaned back and crossed them over my chest. "And it's not like this wheel is taking me anywhere. It's not like I'm going to get to a place. There is no destination. It's all just rote, mechanical movements taking me in a circle. Around and around and around. And there is no joy in it. I lost the joy in it. And I just want it to end. I just want to get off. I want out of it." I reached up to wipe the tears from both of my eyes.

"Then let me help you." My mother held out her hands toward me. "Why won't you ask me for more help? Why won't you tell me what you need?"

I shook my head and bit my lip again. My eyes were closed but the tears escaped them nonetheless.

"Heather, why? Please let me help you. Let *us* help you."

"No," I wept, and then a sob escaped my throat.

"*Why?* We are here to help you—"

"Because I'M THE FUCKUP," I whisper-shouted. "I don't *deserve* your help."

My mother looked from me to Mel and then back to me. She didn't say a word, and then she looked down at her hands in her lap with the sudden realization that this was why Mel wanted her here. She shook her head for a few seconds. "Does she really believe this?" she asked Mel, her eyes still fixed on her own hands.

"This is what she needs most, Linda," Mel answered.

"Heather, you have to know that's not true—"

"Yes, it is." I wouldn't let her finish. "I'm the fuckup. I'm the one who left the church. I'm the one who got fired for her website. I'm the one who got divorced. I'm the one who ends up depressed all the time. I'm the one who can't seem to help herself."

"Oh, Heather . . ." My mother's eyes filled with tears, and she, like me, shut them to try to keep them from pouring down her face. "This just isn't true. This isn't what we feel." She began shaking her head again.

"Heather, you need to tell her why you believe this," Mel said. "She needs to hear it. She needs to hear it from you."

My mother suddenly looked up and over at me. I nodded and my voice cracked as I started speaking. "Do you remember calling me up, back when I was living in that apartment downtown, and telling me that we needed to get lunch? That we needed to talk—"

"Chili's. I asked you to meet me at Chili's," she said. A sad coldness infiltrated her voice.

"Yes, Chili's. You asked me to meet you at Chili's, and over a bowl of chips and salsa you told me that you knew what I was doing, that you were no fool."

A few weeks prior to this meeting at Chili's, at the age of twenty-two, I had moved in with my first boyfriend. He'd been in one of my last English classes at BYU, and even though I experienced no physical attraction to him whatsoever, I'd fallen in love with his brain. He had a photographic memory and loved to dissect issues and problems and spend money that he did not have on computer equipment, stereos, bikes and their accompanying gear, and video games. In fact, instead of using his student loans to pay for graduate school, he bought two giant speakers for his stereo, which in turn he'd bought with the student loan he was supposed to have used to pay for the last semester of his undergraduate degree. I can pick 'em!

In a stadium-sized crowd I can pinpoint the man I will bring into my life only to have to take care of him like a child.

I'd found us a one-bedroom apartment in downtown Salt Lake City, on the third floor of a green brick building next to a Greek Orthodox church, and asked him to move in with me. He wasn't attending his graduate classes anyway, so it just made sense. It made sense for me to move in with an unemployed man-child who was funneling student loan money into a bike he would never ride, who would not ever finish that graduate degree, and who would play online games for twenty hours at a time while I worked two jobs to pay for rent and groceries. But cut me some slack: I was only twenty-two years old and had never had a cup of coffee, because it was against the religion I'd just abandoned. No coffee, no tea, no sex, no kissing with tongue, no R-rated movies. True story: when my brother was serving his Mormon mission in Montreal, Canada, he wrote the family a letter pleading with us to stop watching R-rated films. I was sixteen years old at the time, and my brother was my hero. I'd cried for weeks when he left for that mission, because I wouldn't see him for two years—it has been established that melodrama is my specialty—and when I read that letter, I made a commitment to him, to myself, and most importantly to Our Lord and Savior Jesus Christ that I would not ever watch an R-rated movie again. And I kept that promise for over four years. Four years! Right up until the third of four Matts I would date in college convinced me to watch *Pulp Fiction*. I remember being so traumatized and wondering, *Is this even legal to put in movies now? Is the director in jail?*

My mother knew that I had moved in with my boyfriend, and this was verboten in the Mormon religion. If we'd moved in together, we'd most certainly at some point consummated the relationship:

premarital sex is only one degree less sinful than murder. There was so much that I wanted to tell her as I reached for a tortilla chip. First, that losing my virginity was the most technical and unromantic night of my life, and sex wasn't particularly fun. And second, why hadn't she told me so? Why hadn't she ever told me about urinary tract infections? Why hadn't she ever told me to go pee after having a penis inside of me? Because *of course* I contracted one after that awkwardly technical first time wherein I turned on all the lights and made him lie down and not touch me. All I knew about sex was that it was going to hurt the first time. I knew I would bleed. And I did, quite a bit, but we got it over with. I was so relieved that it was *over* and had no idea that this thing we had just performed could, in fact, be quite pleasurable. Two days later I started peeing fire and had no idea what was going on. I thought I might be dying, and when my roommate at the time heard me screaming in the bathroom, she asked me if I had a UTI.

A what? A UTI? Was that like a UFO?

I didn't have very good insurance, so my boyfriend helped me find a clinic near his place in Provo where I could get tested for a UTI and get a prescription for the pill. How I wished that my mother were the one accompanying me to that appointment; how I longed for her reassuring hand on the back of my head, stroking my hair as I experienced a gynecological exam for the first time. I wanted to tell her that at Chili's, but I didn't. I didn't tell her about the creepy male doctor who, before reaching his hand inside me, said, "We will fix you right up so that every month you are going to know the exact day that you can pop that pad right into your panties!"

"Pop that pad right into your panties." He said those exact words. And to this day, whenever I start my period, I hear him saying that in his disturbing, condescending tone and think about how alone I felt.

I think about the nurse who saw the terror in my eyes and stood in as my mother, who held my hand when the exam became so painful that I burst into silent tears. She squeezed my palm as she asked him to be gentler, and then told me that it would all be over soon. I don't remember her name or even her face, but "It will all be over soon" will go down as one of the most comforting phrases ever uttered to me in my life. I wish my mother had been in that room with me. I missed my mother.

She knew what I was up to. She didn't mention the premarital sex, but she did tell me that she knew I had moved in with my boyfriend. We ate chips and discussed the details of where I lived, what the apartment was like. We also made some small talk about my jobs and my car, my commute and the gas bill, before she finished a chip and became very quiet.

"I need you to know, Heather, that I love you. But without Christ in your life, without Christ in our relationship . . . our relationship can never be the same."

Today my hormonal teenage daughter could tell me that she hates me and it wouldn't even come close in impact to what my mother had just told me. No words will ever be as devastating to me as what she said to me over chips and salsa at Chili's on 400 South in Salt Lake City, Utah.

My very first memory is staring up into my mother's beautiful face as she held me to her chest and breastfed me. I was the only child she breastfed. She thought my father had fallen out of love with her. And because she wanted to be loved—because she was dedicated to remaining with my father, to working it out and honoring the commitment she had made in their temple marriage—she wanted another child.

Me.

I was born to love my mother, and love her I did. She breastfed me for almost two and a half years because I wouldn't eat anything else. In fact, she had to leave the house for an entire weekend to force me to eat solid food. I adored her, followed her everywhere. If I was near her, I was touching her. All of my earliest memories are of her skin and her smell and her touch, the silent way we communicated, the soft way her hair would brush my face when she picked me up, the scent of her neck as I rested my face under her chin, the way I would grip the fold of her skirt as I stood in the kitchen next to her while she stirred a pot for dinner.

I remember being at my brother's soccer game—I must have been three or four at the time, in the late seventies—and a group of mothers were standing around, making small talk. I was gripping my mother's leg like I always did when we were away from the house, out in public: like a baby monkey. When I came out of my daydream only to see my mother standing a few feet away from me, I realized that I had been gripping another woman's leg the whole time. They all laughed when I looked up to see the stranger I'd been holding on to, and she assured me that she didn't mind. But it was exactly like coming out of anesthesia for the first time when I was gripped with panic about piano practice. My mother knew to shush the room, to honor my embarrassment with comfort, not laughter. She rushed to me and swung me into her arms, and the smell of her hair in my face calmed me instantly.

We remained inseparable throughout my childhood, and in the two years leading up to my parents' divorce when I was ten years old our silent communication achieved a new dimension, one filled with shared pain and suffering. I don't think I actively considered the idea of them divorcing, but I felt an impending sense of doom. They fought constantly, relentlessly, and my mother began taking her makeup off in the morning, not at night. I was always there, lingering like a little barnacle. I could always tell that she had been crying. Her eyes with their puffy lids and the bags underneath gave it all away, and I would ask her every morning, "Mom, what's wrong? Why are you sad?"

She would always set down the tissue she was using to wipe the Pond's cold cream from her eyes, reach out her hand to rub the back of my head, and say, "I'm fine. Nothing is wrong." I always wanted to plead with her more, to beg her to tell me, but I was worried that would make her even more emotional. So I accepted her explanation, at least in the sense that I didn't force the issue. But I felt her pain as much as she did; that was the bond we had forged when I was born, through the thirty months I was attached to her breast. And something in my eight-year-old head convinced me that if I didn't cause any trouble—if I made perfect grades and performed better than anyone else in everything that I did—that somehow this would make her happy. This would dry her tears. I would become the valedictorian of kids.

I never told her this, and it was not a burden she put on me. I just wanted my plan to work. And even when it didn't work at first—when they sat us around that square, laminate wood dinner table, my legs squirming on the yellow vinyl of my seat, to tell us that they were getting capital-*D* Divorced—I never stopped believing that one day my plan would work. And eventually it did, of course. Who isn't happy and proud to have a child who makes straight As throughout elementary, middle, and high school? Who wouldn't be happy to have a daughter who is captain of the volleyball team, president of the honor society, recipient of a full scholarship to the college of her choice? Who wouldn't beam while sitting in the audience at high school graduation, listening to her daughter give a speech in front of thousands, because she had not only graduated valedictorian but also with a grade point average higher than anyone else's in the history of the school? Achieving all of that wasn't easy, nor did it make me a particularly fun person to be around. Imagine a wet blanket who argued against the concept of evolution—Mormons don't believe in such nonsense—and threw a tantrum when she missed a single multiple-choice question. Even the nerds wouldn't make eye contact with me.

When I think about that time in my life, sometimes I romanticize it. I want to believe that I was doing it because I was ambitious, because I cared about knowledge and learning and becoming a more realized person. And some of that is true. But I did it more for *her*. Which is why, when she told me over chips and salsa that she and I were not ever going to have what we had had ever again, I felt like she had reached across the table to strangle me. Didn't she know I had done all of that for her? How could she not know that I lived my life for her? I had given her my life.

All I had ever wanted was her, and there she was saying, "I don't want you."

As we sat there with Mel, I told my mother all of this as I twirled the orange tassels of the blanket between my thumb and forefinger. All of it was a bit less coherent and muddled by tears and aching sobs that had spent twenty years in my chest waiting for their moment. I told her that I felt like I had squandered all of that work, that backbreaking and mind-bending work. I had squandered my life's work. All by finally choosing to live for *me*. And she had rejected *me*.

The three of us sat in silence. And then my mother turned to Mel.

"I remember saying that to her; I do," she said. "I did that. And at the time I believed it." Her voice started to tremble when she turned to look at me. "I had no idea that you have been carrying this around all these years, and I am so sorry. *I'm sorry.* I don't feel that way anymore, and I haven't felt that way for a very long time. I know that doesn't make up for any of it, but I hope—"

"It's okay," I interjected. I didn't want her to have to explain anything, and I couldn't possibly have felt more uncomfortable. I know that this is the point of therapy, to lay bare all the bumps and scars and disfigured shapes in us so that we can understand ourselves. But my mother had given so much of herself to me already. She was my main support as a full-time single mother, the one who picked up the phone to listen to me scream. She didn't owe me anything. She really didn't. She had poured blood and sweat and tireless physical energy into the care of my children, and I had no right to ask her for anything.

"Heather," Mel said. "Let her speak."

My mother nodded.

"I love you now as I loved you as a child, perhaps even more. I love your children. I love the way you love your children. And, Heather, I love who you have become, what you have taught me about loving and how to love. I learned through you that I was wrong about how our relationship was supposed to work. Because I cannot deny the love and respect I have for you not only as my daughter but also for the woman you have become. You are you. You are you, and I could not possibly love you more."

Her last sentence was choked as she tried to hold it together. I covered my face with my hands again to hide my tears and vulnerability.

"Please forgive me," she said, and when those words hit my ears, my entire chest jerked with a sob.

I know how lucky I am. I know many people do not have the

privilege of having this kind of relationship with their mother and either desperately wish they did or wish that they were even on speaking terms. I know some of you routinely stab the eyes of a voodoo doll fashioned in the shape of the woman who gave you life, and then you stomp on it and shove it into the garbage disposal. Please don't give Marlo any ideas.

I am lucky, and I don't ever take this gift for granted. She is the most generous and loving mother a human being could ever hope for, and I am the one who got her. I am the fuckup who scored her.

Now that we had *that* little chips-and-salsa misunderstanding cleared up, it was time to make a plan. Mel whipped out a pencil and pad of paper. I thought about making a joke about smartphones with apps that render list making and sharing quite easy, but my mother had just made an apology I didn't know that I needed to hear and an entire chamber of my heart had instantly healed. I could shut my mouth for once.

"Two days a week. You need to give her two days," Mel stated, and I nearly fell off the sofa.

"No!" I yelled. "You cannot ask her to do that. Not two days."

"Why not? It's just two days, Heather. We are not asking your mother for a kidney, although clearly she'd give you one."

"Because you don't know my mother's life!" My mother retired from Avon to spend more time with my sister's five kids and my brother's five kids and my two kids and my stepfather's four grandchildren. That's, like, 5,000 people she has to love, and she doesn't show love like some normal person. My mother is the valedictorian of showing love, and when she is not clocking steps around her living room, she is taking care of grandchildren. There's this joke that my siblings and I tell each other, except it's less of a joke and more of a bitch session. It's about the relationship my mother forges with each of our children, how at some point during the first three years of each child's life they will—and there have been zero exceptions to this—cry out at night for Grandmommy. Not for Mom or Dad or even Santa Claus. *Grandmommy*. And the only way to retaliate is to call her at whatever ungodly hour it is to say, "SHE WANTS YOU." Except my mother does not process this as retaliation. She relishes it.

"I can give her two days," my mother said.

"That's too mu—"

"I WILL BE GIVING YOU TWO DAYS. So, laundry, dishes . . ."

"Can you help her with her grocery shopping?" asked Mel.

"Absolutely. And we'll help the girls get showered on those days as well. We'll come and get the chores done as the girls are finishing up homework and then we'll make dinner and help get them to bed. I don't know why I didn't think of this sooner. Thank you, Mel."

Mel was scribbling on her notepad as fast as she could. After underlining something twice, she looked up at me with a smirk.

"Was that so hard?" she asked. "How much money have you spent in here having me tell you to ask her for help? You could have bought a boat, Heather. And now your mom's going to be washing your underwear."

That was the plan we made—two days a week. Mel also made me promise that I wouldn't protest if my mother offered even more help. Didn't I know how lucky I was that she was my mother? I mean, with such a wonderful mother, one wouldn't think I could get so depressed. However, depression like this is just as unmoved by a wonderful mother as it is by a long, hot shower. And so, in honor of every other parent out there struggling to do all of this by themselves—every other parent scrambling to hold it all together, all while meeting deadlines and paying bills and not running out of gas on the way to parent-teacher conferences or play practice, and, yes, the backdoor needs a weather strip and the kitchen faucet is leaking—we will get to those things after we get to the book report and the science fair project and talking our child down from an existential hormonal crisis. We have only two hands and we do this all alone, every day, again and again and again. On behalf of those of us who didn't score my mother, I promised I would accept her help.

ELEVEN
PLENTY OF FISH

THE CALL TIME FOR every treatment seemed to run later and later, and they didn't need me to come in for my fourth treatment until 2:00 p.m. on a Wednesday. This would mean another twenty hours without food, so by pure accident I had begun practicing a form of "intermittent fasting." I don't want to dismiss it as a fad diet, given the testimonies I've read and heard from people who believe it has changed their lives; but after the marathon was over and I couldn't lose the ten pounds I'd gained while training for it, I was desperate for some solution. A friend told me about intermittent fasting: some people fast for sixteen hours a day, others fast for an entire twenty-four-hour period twice a week. It's supposed to help with weight loss and sharpen your memory and lengthen your life span. I tried the sixteen-hour variation and lasted a week. I thought about food constantly. I was ravenous, and when you take food away from someone who (a) cannot stop thinking about food, and

(b) wants to be dead, that person will become even more obsessed with food.

In the seven days since I had started the treatment, though, I'd lost two or three pounds. I broke out a pair of jeans I hadn't worn in over eighteen months and paired it with something other than a T-shirt, something that looked like it might have been ironed. I woke up an hour early to shower knowing that I had a weekly team meeting with the nonprofit shortly after I'd be getting home from dropping the girls off at school. I even put on a little bit of makeup. There was something about the idea of being around all these technicians and nurses and doctors who were performing something so, well, *intimate* on me that I started to feel like I needed to show up a bit. Like I needed them to know how much I appreciated what they were doing, what they were attempting. Walking in without trailing body odor seemed like a good place to start.

When my mother and stepfather showed up at 1:00 p.m.—yes, nearly an hour early—to head up to the clinic, I was in my bedroom putting on a necklace and a couple of gold bracelets. My mother called out to me and found me standing in front of the mirror in my bedroom, fastening the clasp on my necklace. She gasped.

"What's wrong?" I asked.

"Heather, you look *stunning*," she said. She'd placed her hands over her chest to brace herself.

"Aw, you're being really nice. You have to say that because you're my mom."

"No, really. You look so lovely in that outfit." My outfit? Straight, solid-colored jeans, a white blouse made out of a fabric that looked like it had been ironed when in fact it needed no ironing at all, black boots that laced all the way to the top. She was right. It was an *outfit*. I hadn't worn an outfit in . . . weeks? Months? I'd literally worn nothing but yoga pants, sports bras, and T-shirts for so long that I couldn't remember ever thinking about what shoes would go best. I was always wearing my running shoes or flip-flops because I didn't have to think about those. And the exhaustion of thinking about it is what prevented me from wearing anything that would require thinking in the first place. But I really hadn't thought about it much that morning. I knew I had to get up early, I knew I had to shower—HOLY GOD. I had taken a shower and I hadn't grabbed at my torso in disgust.

"I took a shower, Mom, and I didn't hate it," I blurted upon the realization. "Isn't that weird? Like, I'm *glad* I showered." She started to chuckle. "If this whole thing doesn't work, at least I'll be clean for three weeks. The study may be free but I'm going to have to buy more shampoo."

As we climbed into the minivan my stomach audibly growled, and yet I wasn't really bothered by it. I was hungry, yes, but I wasn't ravenous. I wasn't thinking about food or the next meal I would eat. The last seven days had forced my attention elsewhere: Would this work? Would I ever feel better? Were we wasting our time? Would I ever not want to be dead? This was all I thought about now, because if this didn't work, what then? And I tried not to go past the "then" into the various scenarios, which of course ended up with me living homeless and alone.

I walked ahead of my mother and stepfather into the waiting room at the clinic. As I headed straight for Greg and his clipboard of questions, a staff member named Lauren walked around the front desk. I never knew what color her hair was going to be on any given day: sometimes it was pink but that day it was purple and she was wearing a black-and-white polka-dot dress with opaque silver tights. I have always had such admiration for people who can dress like this, who can bear the attention of the people they know and don't know analyzing their wardrobes.

Lauren stopped me before I could get to the desk and grabbed my right arm.

"You have the most amazing clothes!" she said, assessing me from head to toe. "Like, I love to see what you're going to wear each time you're here. It just keeps getting better."

I almost fell over. This was the last thing I ever expected to hear from anyone ever in my life, especially from a person who could pull off the most outrageous combinations of clothes.

"Oh my God," I stammered. "That's one of the nicest things anyone has ever said to me. I . . . just . . . thank you."

"I'm taking notes!" she added.

"So am I! I mean, look at your legs. Those tights!"

"Oh, these old things? I have them in every color of the rainbow. I was feeling the silver this morning." She patted me on my arm and continued past me so she could attend to her administrative work. Just then my mother leaned over to whisper in my ear.

"Is she the most adorable thing, or what?"

That was something so remarkable about this place, the ease with which everyone interacted with each other and with the patients and with those who accompanied the patients. It didn't feel clinical or medicinal or fraught with the weight of *Here is where we shock people into seizures.*

Everything from that point forward proceeded as usual. We waited about a half hour after I filled out the Just How Depressed Are You? questionnaire (still really, really depressed), and then Molly and I chatted about the myth of cranberry juice and its supposed magical effects on UTIs as she struggled to get the needle into my right arm. Still hadn't had sex! What would it be like to want to get naked with someone? Bare skin touching someone else's bare skin? Who does that? Gross. Stop. Don't even get a room; just occupy yourselves otherwise.

When I walked back into the waiting room after the needle insertion, I nodded at my mother to indicate that it had been awful yet again, and she took hold of my arms as I sat down beside her.

She looked at the bruises in both arms and shook her head. "There has to be a better way of doing this, right? Why are they making this so painful?"

"I don't think it's their fault," I said, wanting to take Molly's side. "They aren't used to these needles. And, my God, if this is the most painful part of this procedure, I think we are walking away with the bank."

Only a few minutes passed before they called me in, and I crossed the hallway into the room toward my gurney.

"Heather B. Armstrong. July nineteenth, 1975," I answered before the nurse could even ask me. And before I knew it I was awake, propped up in the gurney, and being rolled into the recovery room. It had gone by *that fast*. A blip, like someone had snapped their fingers. I remember the vial of propofol, the Velcro, and the wire, but who was the anesthesiologist? I . . . I couldn't . . . *Jesus Christ, my eyes!*

"Who stabbed my eyes? Was it you?" I yelled at a nurse I couldn't recognize. "Why did you stab me in the eyes? Why would you do this?"

"I'm sorry, do your eyes hurt?" he asked, his voice professionally gentle.

"Do they hurt?" I drunkenly shot back at him. "Didn't I just say that you stabbed me? Why would I say that if they didn't hurt? Why would you do this? Was it you?"

I blinked several times and then frantically looked for my mother. When I found her across the room, reaching into the tiny fridge to grab me a cup of apple juice, I blinked a few more times and asked, "Were you there the whole time? You didn't leave me, did you?"

She quickly turned around and rushed to my side. "Of course I didn't leave you. I was there the whole time. In fact, they let me take some pictures of the abyss!"

I ignored her enthusiasm, at least temporarily, because of the agonizing pain in my eyes. "Did you see if my eyes were closed? Were my eyes closed?"

"I'm sure they were," she answered. "I watched you go under, your hands falling to your sides."

"My eyes hurt like . . . I can't explain it—"

"We can ask the team to tape your eyes shut from now on," the nurse offered, even though I had just brazenly accosted him. "Sometimes your eyelids can drift open a bit when you're under. We'll make sure this doesn't happen again."

I was still feeling drunk, so I laid my head back against the gurney, shut my eyes, and began to make a list of what my chart must look like: allergic to fentanyl, becomes constipated by something unknown, must tape eyelids shut. This list fanned out my many charms as well as my online dating profiles, which was yet another reason I'd ended up wanting to be dead.

The dating scene in Utah is a beautiful backdrop for a suicidal ideation.

I'd been in two long-distance relationships after my divorce. Both times I realized the mileage between us was untenable, given the demands of my kids and my job. Sure, sex can be really great when you haven't seen someone in six weeks, but during those six weeks I still only had two hands and needed to unload the dishwasher, fold four loads of laundry, help my kid with the Pythagorean theorem, build a robot for the science fair, take my kids to the dentist, volunteer for the bake sale, and somewhere in there make enough money to pay rent and buy food and put gas in the car. Those romances were more like fantasy vacations than actual relationships. Then I made the horrible mistake of deciding that I should try to date men who lived within a day's driving distance from my house. This ended up being one of the worst mistakes of my entire life.

While training for the Boston Marathon, I set up an account on Match.com. What on earth was I thinking? It just seemed more adult than swiping through Tinder because I was not looking to hook up or date casually. I did not have time for that trivial nonsense. I had no interest in that kind of dating, since I never took a lunch break and hadn't had time to grab a cup of coffee with a friend since my kids' father moved across the country and I got primary custody of my children. *Since then.*

I did have a Tinder account, and a Bumble account, and eventually I signed up for an account on a site called Plenty of Fish. I kept it open for the specific purpose of being able to reference it in case I ever needed to prove to someone just how terrorizing the dating pool is for women in Utah. It may be just as terrorizing for men—I mean, look at me! Have you met me? I'm so crazy, I agreed to let a doctor flatline my brain ten times! Also, one should note that I will at some point want to have rough picnic bench sex with someone else, although I did fail to disclose that in any of my profiles. What I did eventually end up writing in every profile I had was "The fish that you caught or the deer that you shot do not matter to me as much as the words coming out of your mouth." Because, holy shit, y'all, the photos of dead animals in the dating profiles of men in Utah . . . And, my God, do not even think of setting up a dating profile, dude in Utah, unless you have a shot of yourself in full gear on the top of a slope at Alta Ski Area, or you will not be getting *any* in the near future. Any of what, I'm not sure.

I just opened my Plenty of Fish account, and underneath the heading "These people are more likely to respond to your messages— start having more conversations now!" is a photo of a man straddling a dead moose. He is straddling it, the moose that is dead. And, OH MY GOD, I just looked at the rest of the photos in his profile and you will never guess. He's holding not one, not two, not even three dead fish. He is holding *six* dead fish. Plenty!

I have tried to be very careful about dating and relationships around my children, and once in the summer of 2015 while vacation- ing in Southern California with a large group of friends Leta sensed that I had become attracted to a certain bachelor I'd just met. She noticed him touching my arm and I spent the next hour alone with her on a twin bed at a condo overlooking the Palm Desert assuring her that I wasn't going to fall in love with a man and leave her. She was terrified that I'd get into a relationship with someone who didn't live in Utah and move. And *leave* her. She was afraid that I'd up and leave her and Marlo. Where she conjured up this notion *we will never know*, but her reaction was visceral and almost primal. I'd always known to be careful about introducing the men in my life to my children—I dated the jealous man for over eighteen months before he met my kids—but this response from her made me even more cautious.

However, when I set up my Match.com account and began look- ing at profiles, I stumbled across one that I had to share with Leta, only because I knew that we could laugh about it together. Someone set up a profile and in every picture he was standing on his head. He was on top of a famous mountain, standing on his head. He was in the middle of a lake on a paddleboard, standing on his head. He was in the crowd at a baseball game, a hot dog in each hand, standing on his head. He was in a dark cave surrounded by human skulls, standing on his head. I suppose he thought women would find this witty, or I guess we were supposed to be impressed by his head-standing skills. But if you show me a picture of yourself in an awkward pose surrounded by human skulls, on purpose, I am not ever going to take my clothes off in front of you.

I went on so many first dates, I'm not sure I can even count that high, and only a handful of times went on a second date. I once agreed to a second date even though I was in no way attracted to the man. But he had a great job. A man with a stable job! What would that be like to date someone who could help pay the bills? He was a pediatric psychologist, so I knew he could afford groceries. On that second date, after I had rearranged my life in order to leave my house—finishing up homework with both kids, overseeing piano practice, hiring a babysitter, making sure the babysitter knew Marlo's bedtime routine, making sure I'd prepared a meal for both kids, tying up all loose ends with work, making sure the dog had been fed and let outside, all while taking a dreaded shower and spending the time to style my hair and apply makeup—that pediatric psychologist told me over a table of steaming Indian food that I was using my children as an excuse to make men think I was unattainable.

I know it sounds like I'm complaining, and that's because I am. I have my kids all day every day, week in and week out, and in order to go on a date with a man I had to navigate the reality of this. Yet, every single man I went on a date with either didn't have children or shared custody with his ex. He could simply shower and walk out the door. I grappled with the inevitable resentment I felt at this glaring, blinding disparity. The pediatric psychologist and I had had to reschedule the second date because Marlo had gotten sick hours before, and apparently he thought I had made up that inconvenience to manipulate him. Yes, I am one to avoid conflict like the plague and will endure a lot of bullshit because of the PTSD of being cornered against a wall. But I let down my guard, set down my fork, and leaned closer to him to say, "I took a fucking shower for you." And then I got up and walked out. I walked away from a bowl of aloo gobi, a plate of chana masala, and two giant samosas, if you can imagine.

I went on so many dates with men who talked about their carefree lives or complained endlessly about their exes. And never once did a guy offer to pay for a meal or a drink. Not once. My resentment built with each weak cocktail and soy latte, and I really did believe I was going to live the rest of my life alone. The tedious maneuvers of this ongoing ritual, despite seeing someone novel every week—and not one offering even a whiff of romance—left me feeling completely alone.

And so, when someone did actually engage in the tiniest amount of flirting—before our first date he asked me about my job and shared that he taught kayaking lessons at a local college, and I was so desperate I convinced myself he was flirting—I jumped at the idea that we might go beyond a second date. And we did. We went on a third and fourth and fifth date, and because he was really attractive and nicer than Mr. Rogers, I ignored the fact that we did not agree on any political matter. I ignored the fact that he did not vote in the presidential election. I ignored the fact that I was vegan and he routinely hunted deer. I ignored the fact that he described in detail the fifteen different guns he had stockpiled in his basement. I also ignored the fact that he did not ever want to be intimate with me. I shoehorned myself into that relationship and suppressed my very essence merely because he had asked me about my job. He ran his own business and loved his son, and so I resisted reaching out to touch him lovingly because, even after six weeks, he had never initiated physical contact. But I could make it work, I thought. I convinced myself that I could live like that. Because what man would ever flirt with me again? This had to work, and if it didn't, I would be alone forever. Add this to the list of things you should know about people who suffer from depression: we are lonely and we fear that this loneliness is our destiny. We despise this loneliness—we certainly don't want to feel alone and are not choosing to feel alone—but we feel it desperately, wholly, all-consumingly. We think we will be alone forever.

After a Mexican dinner one night during the week of Christmas—a week I'd been dreading because my children would be with their father and I would be spending the holiday without them—he and I returned to my empty house. When he plopped himself on my couch, perched his feet on my coffee table, and clasped his hands behind his head with a sigh of relaxation, I suddenly realized, *Oh my God, we are not ever going to be intimate. He is not sexually attracted to me. How can I possibly live like this? Do I want to be in a relationship with someone who does not find me attractive? Can I live with that?* And the pressure of trying to hold it all together, my children 2,200 miles across the country and waking up on Christmas morning without me—my God, that pain—it made me sit on the opposite side of the couch and put my head in my hands. I couldn't hold back the pain any longer and it started to pour out of my eyes. He immediately pulled his feet off of the table and put his hands into his lap, sitting upright. Instead of saying anything, he just shook his head, and that reaction made me cry even harder.

Finally he broke his silence. "Do you have something to tell me?" he asked.

I shrugged my shoulders almost unnoticeably. "I don't know," I muttered. And then, without any thought or reason, I said, "Maybe you should leave." It wasn't what I wanted to say; it just came out of my mouth involuntarily.

He stood up, walked over to me, and stood a foot away. "Is that what you really want?" he asked.

I couldn't form words at that point: the pain and the confusion and the fear of being alone were compressing my chest. I felt like someone had taken a vise and was using it to crush my lungs.

He walked past me, grabbed his coat from the back of the couch, and headed toward the front door. When I heard his steps on the Spanish tiles in the hallway leading to the foyer, I rushed to him and grabbed his arm just as he reached the door.

"Please don't leave," I cried. "Please. That's not what I want." Here I was pleading with a man who did not know me, the *real* me, who could never understand the depth of my plea and why my heart and my body and my brain were in such conflict. "Please," I begged once more.

He shook his head, gently pulled my hand away from his arm, and walked out the door without saying a word. When he closed the door behind him, I immediately fell to the floor in a heap. I pulled my arms over my head and rocked back and forth on my knees, and then I started howling. Wild, aching howls erupted from my body interspersed with screaming.

"I don't want to feel this way anymore!" I yelled. I was alone again, alone forever. "Make it stop, please make it stop, please *make it stop!*" I pleaded over and over again. I felt an eerie darkness, a cold and dangerous darkness, start to wrap itself around me as if it were going to reach up and strangle me. I was terrified. Scared of that darkness and of the thoughts thunderously clouding my head. Somehow I crawled around the corner of the foyer over those cold Spanish tiles to the phone on the edge of the countertop in the kitchen and dialed my mother's phone number. She picked up as a howl escaped my throat.

"Heather, where are you?" she asked, the fear in her voice matching the fear that had enveloped me.

"Please make it stop!" I wailed.

"Make what stop? Make what stop, Heather?"

"I don't want to feel this way anymore!"

"What happened?" she pleaded. "Tell me what happened."

"It doesn't matter what happened; I will always feel this way and I just want to be dead."

"Heather—"

"If I am dead, I won't feel this way anymore!"

"We are getting in the car right now and we are coming to be with—"

"Please make it stop!"

"Do not put down the phone, Heather. Listen to me. *Listen. To. Me.* Do not put down the phone—"

"I will never stop feeling this way, Mom. Please make it stop."

"You are going to talk to me until I get to your front door and you are going to let me in, okay? Do you understand me?" She didn't sound threatening or judgmental. She sounded like a commander laying out a battle plan. "Talk to me. Where are you in the house?"

"I'm in the kitchen. On the floor."

"What part of the kitchen?"

"I'm next to the pantry."

This small talk continued for the entire forty-minute drive from her house to mine, and then I heard the knock at my front door both in the house and through the phone. I walked to the foyer, and when I opened the door we both had phones pressed to our ears. I hung up and dropped my hand to my side and just fell into her chest like a two-year-old needing her mother.

"Please make it stop," I mumbled one last time. My stepfather walked in and passed us as he headed upstairs to my bedroom.

"Rob is going to turn your bed down and I am going to walk you up there and stay with you until you fall asleep, okay?"

"You know I don't ever make my bed, Mom. There is nothing to turn down." Somehow, in the midst of all that pain, the warmth of her chest had given me the strength to inject some small bit of levity into one of the scariest moments of my life.

"Do not argue with me, young lady," she shot back. "We brought clothes and are going to sleep in your guest room, okay?" I nodded and she reached for my hand and led me to my bed. Since I had actually dressed up for this date, I excused myself to my bathroom, yanked off my pants and shirt, and grabbed my bathrobe. When I walked back into my bedroom, she was sitting at the foot of the giant king-sized bed where I slept alone every night. She patted the mattress next to her, an indication that I should not argue and that I needed to get some sleep. She was right: I needed to sleep off this darkness.

I walked over, sat down, and grabbed my giant bag of pills. After getting each one out for the night and swallowing them, I climbed underneath my covers. My mother pulled my duvet up to my neck and tucked it up under my ears.

"Tomorrow we are going to call your psychiatrist—"

"Mom, no. You know we can't."

"Do not argue with me. I am going to dial his number for you and stand next to you while you make an appointment. If you don't make the appointment, I will. We will do this together. We will make this stop."

"But what if—"

"But nothing. We will call him tomorrow morning. Now get some rest." She reached up and stroked my hair along my forehead down to my shoulder just like I do with Leta when she is feeling anxious or uneasy. I always wanted to be the mom that my mom was to me.

The meds kicked in immediately—they always did—which was another reason I had not wanted to call my psychiatrist. My meds still helped me fall asleep. I didn't want that to change.

The following morning I lingered in my anxiety a little longer than usual. Since the girls were spending the week with their father, I didn't have to perform the morning routine. When I finally made it downstairs in a dirty T-shirt and yoga pants, my mother was standing in the kitchen, holding my landline. I was about to protest when she held up her hand.

"I don't think his office is open just yet. It's not even eight o'clock," I said.

"You can leave a message and tell them to call you back."

I pulled out my iPhone to look up his office phone number, and then I took the landline out of my mother's hand.

I slowly dialed Dr. Bushnell's office. I don't know why the movement of my fingers held such gravity. I had purposefully not called him because I believed that in doing so Jon would find out. Something about getting Dr. Bushnell's help—the help I so clearly needed—meant that Jon would know I was this depressed. The idea that he might use this against me was terrifying.

After I dialed the last number, I held the phone to my ear and heard his line immediately go to voicemail. The rush of relief made my entire body heave.

"Hey, Stacy. This is Heather Armstrong. I know I haven't seen Dr. Bushnell in a while, but I need a refill on my Valium and they told me I needed to call you guys about it. If you could give me a call back, I'd really appreciate it."

I was not lying. This was all true. I had three days' worth of Valium left—a critical component of the cocktail of medication that treated my insomnia—and my pharmacy had told me that they'd tried to call my doctor for a refill and were given strict orders that I needed to call him myself. We know why now, but at the time I was, like, *Does no one understand?* Making time to see a doctor on top of having to do one more goddamn load of laundry was just too much.

Stacy called back within the hour and informed me that Dr. Bushnell was traveling until the end of January, so we scheduled that fateful appointment for February on Leta's birthday. She kindly called in a prescription for enough pills to get me through the month, and then ended with "He really, really wants to see you."

And *see* me he did. Thank God he saw me.

TWELVE
DEAR FAMILY AND FRIENDS

AFTER I WOKE UP from being dead for the fourth time, berated that
innocent nurse for my dry eyes, and argued for more than ten minutes about why it was 1979, my parents drove me home. We stopped
at the Asian market two blocks away to pick up some poop tea. I
still hadn't gone to the restroom. In addition to my dry eyes, I was
starting to have stomach cramps. My grandmother, Geneva Boone—
we called her Granny Boone—had lived with my mother and my
stepfather in the ten years leading up to her death, and she drank
poop tea every single night of those ten years. She'd grown up during
the Depression and kept empty butter and sour cream containers
underneath her bed. She washed out ziplock bags and reused them
dozens of times. I knew this was a common habit of people who had
endured the poverty of those years, but it had never dawned on me
that perhaps they endured crippling constipation from having little
to no nutritious food.

The treatment had gone so late that we didn't pull into my drive-way until after 5:00 p.m., but my mother said that this would be perfect timing. I'd drink the tea with some food like Granny did every night and by the following morning everything would be working again. She assured me of this—everything would be working again—and as she boiled some water on the stove she turned to me and said, "Let it steep for about an hour even though it says only two minutes on the box. The box doesn't know what it's talking about. I'm going to go start a load of laundry."

She and my stepfather still helped out twice a week like Mel had asked them to do. The kids were finishing up homework with the babysitter, so I had about fifteen minutes to go to my room and be alone. That's all I wanted at that moment. Something about the emp-tiness of my stomach, the simultaneous hunger and lack of hunger, made me want to curl up and hide my head under a pillow, even if it was for just fifteen minutes. I didn't want to eat anything. I just wanted to be with myself in the quiet, comforting darkness of my bedroom.

In the eighteen months that I'd burrowed into this hole, I hadn't ever come close to hurting myself. I hadn't ever tried to take my own life. There, I finally said the words out loud. *Take my own life.* Suicide. I had not thought about ways that I would do it if the pain ever became too unbearable. I had during previous depressive epi-sodes thought about the means and the tools I'd use. Even though these eighteen months had been the worst of my life, I knew that my children needed me despite the overwhelming and nauseating belief that they would be better off without me. My responsibility to them, especially given how close we had grown as a family unit of three, barricaded my brain from ever wandering into thoughts of pills or razors or Google searches about how to buy a gun in Utah.

And I was very well aware of this roadblock. I knew that I would not ever attempt to take my life, although I wanted nothing more than to be dead. The irony was not lost on me. And because I knew, I never once thought to write a note. *A note*. "Hey family, your mother/daughter/sister is dead, but here's this piece of paper to remember her by! It's got some words on it. Be nice to each other as you fight over all her clothes."

As I lay in my bed with my head buried under my pillow, I thought about this idea of a note. I had not ever read a suicide note, maybe because I did not want to be confronted with the reflection of myself in the words of someone who'd ended their own life. And not because I am judgmental about that—how could I be? I know the pain; I understand the pain. I had lived the pain every second of every hour of every day for over eighteen months. That is why I cannot and will not ever accuse someone who has killed themselves of being selfish. Is it tragic? Absolutely. It is tragic that the human brain can convince someone to believe that the world would be a better and brighter place without their soul inside it. That is the lie of a suicidal ideation: that our beautiful bodies and minds and gifts to this world are instead a scourge upon it. How were we ever so stupid to believe that we had the right to take up space?

I could not fathom having enough paper to write what I would want to say before removing my life from the lives of those I love so dearly. No one who has been spared this kind of pain would understand why I was gone, so why would I offer reasons? Do you take up space in a note with the lies of your depression, or do you instead save that space for expressions of gratitude? Gratitude, however, implies that you know your life is worth something, so why did you do it? If you had such love for your children, why are you gone? None of it would make sense. A note does not make sense. The only way a note would make sense is if it read, "I am a rat bastard who wants you to suffer." That would be a reason people could wrap their heads around. If the note admits to selfishness, then it would make all the sense in the world. Saying that I love my children so much that I could no longer ignore the truth that their lives would be better if I was not in it? That made sense to no one but me.

I have been writing about both of my children since their births—stories of their infancy and toddlerhood and the rigorous triumphs and blows of motherhood. I have often thought that if anything ever happened to me, that my children would have all these words I have written about them and to them and for them to pore over in my absence. They'd know just how much I loved them in the notes I had been writing their entire lives. And yet, if something did ever happen to me, wouldn't they have wanted a chance to say goodbye? And would the lack of that parting gesture haunt them in greater proportion due to the love they'd feel through my writing? Is this why people write suicide notes? Because even though we know no one will understand, at least a goodbye was spoken? Like, *This is what I can offer you*? How does that make any sense?

And yet, when someone takes their life and doesn't leave a note, we scream, "*Why, why, why? Why* did they do this?" Couldn't they have at least offered the warmth of that parting gesture? As if that note could possibly make sense to anyone but the deceased.

This parting gesture was another reason I did not come close to hurting myself. I would not ever want to leave my children without spending hours and weeks retelling stories and reliving memories, and in continuing to live I was permanently inside of that gesture. I had just reconciled myself to the fact that I would not ever feel better, that I would not ever remember what it felt like to want to be alive. I would not ever sit down and write, "Dear Family, I know you don't understand and I don't expect you to. But I know your lives will be easier with the space that I am leaving you. I am no longer your burden."

I found myself crying when I thought of that word—"burden"—because that's exactly what I had become. The ongoing, ceaseless fuckup. But I needed to rein it in, pull myself out from underneath my pillow, and relieve my babysitter for the night. The light from the kitchen burned my dry eyes as I ascended the stairs from my basement bedroom.

"Are you okay, Mom?" Marlo asked with obvious concern. She was sitting at the kitchen countertop, watching a *Minecraft* video on her iPad. I hadn't eaten in almost twenty hours and I had just composed a brief suicide note in my head that I won't ever really write, but that's what my brain does sometimes. I'm not ever going to feel better, and occasionally I try to articulate and sort through that feeling so that I can figure out how to get up tomorrow morning to do it all again, All of the Things Needing to Get Done.

"I'm fine," I lied. Then I turned to Lyndsey. "Thank you for all your help today. And every day. I couldn't do this without you."

"You feeling any better?" she asked, genuinely concerned.

"Well . . ." I trailed off a bit. "Better is relative, isn't it? Let's just say that I'm not giving up on it yet." She nodded, grabbed her purse, and said goodbye to Marlo and to my stepfather, who was sitting on the couch, waiting for my mother to finish that load of laundry.

I hadn't given up on it yet. Not yet. I was pinning the only hope I'd felt in eighteen months on something in which I didn't believe: miracles.

THIRTEEN

A NEEDLE INTO THE PERFECT GROOVE

FRIDAY, MARCH 17, 2017. St. Patrick's Day. The clinic had called me the day before to inform me I was scheduled for 1:00 the following afternoon. I don't remember much about it being St. Patrick's Day other than Marlo assuring me and Leta that no one could pinch her because she was wearing two green hair ties around her right wrist.

We'd found a shirt that morning in her dresser that had a green flower on it, too, so she talked endlessly about her green items on the drive to school: if anyone pinched her, she'd drag them to the principal and very much like a lawyer she'd prove her case. I was listening to her, sort of, but couldn't really get my mind off my stomach and the knots that were tying it up and pulling in agonizing directions. I'd drunk the poop tea two nights previously, an hour after I'd let it begin steeping. And then . . . nothing. Nothing happened. When I called my mother the next afternoon to tell her that nothing was happening, I managed to pull off something no one has ever accomplished: I made her speechless. She stopped talking for a full ten seconds. I almost hung up and called an ambulance in case she'd stopped breathing.

"But no one can outsmart poop tea," she finally said incredulously. "Perhaps you just need to give it some more time."

"I'm not trying to *outsmart* poop tea, Mom. I want it to work. It's been over eighteen hours since I drank it. It should have worked by now, right?"

"Yes, it should have woken you up this morning, in fact. We have to bring this up with the doctors tomorrow."

"Oh God. No. We are not bringing up outsmarting poop tea in front of Dr. Mickey, no—"

"Heather, this is serious. How many days has it been?"

"Ten." *It has been ten days.* Who goes ten days? *Me.* I go ten days, that's who. This is just beautiful irony that right when I finally gain the maturity and insight to start finding talk of poop unsettling, *I have to talk about poop.*

"They need to know this for their research—"

"I do not want my poop to be part of their research!"

When we ended our conversation, I had a sinking feeling that proved prophetic. When we walked into the clinic at 1:00 p.m. on St. Patrick's Day and I grabbed the clipboard to sign my Just How Awful Do You Feel About Yourself Today? papers, my mother leaned over the counter and whispered to Greg, "We really need to talk to the doctors today about Heather's bowel movements"—as if Greg must adhere to a chain of custody that required him to pass along any information about my poop. Also, can we just acknowledge how awful a euphemism "bowel movement" is?

This would be my fifth treatment. Almost halfway through. I filled out the paperwork with answers almost identical to the ones I'd given ten days previously, before they ever tried to stick that oversized needle into my arm. When I finished the questionnaire, I slumped into the seat next to my mother and leaned to rest my head on my mother's shoulder. She was telling some story about one of my nieces or nephews, I can't remember which one—you can't expect anyone in a Mormon family to remember how many nieces and nephews they have—and I was just too tired to arrange what was coming out of her mouth into any coherent narrative. About fifteen minutes later they called me back for needle prep, where I was happy to see Molly.

"Oh, thank God, it's you," I said as I slid into my place next to all the supplies. She'd been preparing for me, so the gear was already laid out.

"Oh yeah? Well, it's good to see you, too!"

"No, I mean it. It's not like anyone here is bad at what they do. It's just that . . . I don't know. Coming here . . . doing this . . . you find comfort in certain things, and you're part of that for me. Also, to save you some time: still no action in the sack. They should officially reinstate my virginity."

She laughed with her whole chest. "I totally get it. And I'm sorry we're all still getting the hang of these needles." After entering in all the information concerning my meds, she tied a tourniquet around the top of my left arm and had me hang it off the side of the chair into a straighter line. It would be the first and only time someone would get the needle all the way in on the initial try.

"See!" I said. When I looked down to see the needle hanging out of my arm, I realized just how bruised and beat-up I looked. Brown and yellow clouds bloomed from injection sites three to four inches in both directions, the colors so saturated that it looked as if someone had clubbed me with a hammer. Molly could see me inspecting the carnage and apologized again.

"Really, we aren't usually this bad at our jobs," she said. "This specific needle, though, is just a lot harder to wrangle than what we're used to."

"I'm okay," I said. "In fact, there's something about these bruises that feels emblematic of this whole experience. There really isn't an outward manifestation of going through all of this. I know there doesn't have to be, but I see these wounds and realize that I'm actively *doing something* about the last eighteen months of my life instead of screaming obscenities into the phone with my Mormon mother on the other end."

She nodded and suddenly I felt a little exposed. "Sorry," I said. "I know you're not my therapist. I just had that realization sitting here."

"Don't apologize," she offered. "We are here to help, and sometimes that help takes very different shapes and forms."

"Thank you," I said. And I meant that. It takes a village to raise kids, right? And I had my village to help me with that. It also felt like I had another village here to help me get better, and I'd started to want to get better not just for me and my kids but for these people, too—for the doctors and nurses and assistants. I wanted them to feel that they were good at what they do, because they were. They were so good to me.

After Molly wrapped some paper tape around the needle, I returned to the waiting room only to find Dr. Mickey sitting next to my mother, the two of them deep in conversation. Oh God. I was certain she was talking to him about *that*. And I was right. As I took the seat next to my stepfather I heard her say, "Ten days. I mean, that's unheard-of, right?"

Please let me be dead if only because two people who were not me were talking about my poop.

He nodded at my mother's question, scratched his head, and paused for just a few moments. "You know, some of these drugs have side effects that happen so infrequently that the documentation on them is lacking. We'll definitely research all the possibilities." He then looked at me and smiled, as if saying words to me was too much and he wanted to offer me dignity. He got up, straightened his suit, and told us it'd be another few minutes: they were getting the room ready for me. When he turned to leave, I remember looking at the wooden arm of my chair, the blond curve of it. I remember wanting to memorize the way the rows of chairs were arranged, one along the opposite side of the room, another perpendicular to that, below a giant window.

There were two rows of chairs in the middle of the room, one facing the window overlooking the corridor leading to the entrance of the building, the other facing the check-in desk. I studied the fabric on the backs and the seats and traced the lines in the pattern with my eyes. Then I looked up at the fluorescent lighting dotting the ceiling, the way it left some parts of the room darker than others. I wanted to remember all of it, because I knew that I was one of only a few who would get to sit there in that room waiting to walk across the hall to have my brain manipulated by an anesthesiologist. I was just the third patient in this study. Dr. Bushnell had not violated anyone's privacy when he looked at me over the tops of his glasses to emphasize the gravity of his words when he said, "There have been two before you. And you? I have no doubt that this is the answer."

Just then a research assistant walked in and asked, "You ready?" Then she gestured for us to follow her. The three of us stood up from the wooden chairs, in the row along the south side of the room underneath a different window, one that looked out toward the room where the phlebotomists wrestled with the 22-gauge needle. We all walked across the hall into the room where my gurney awaited me. After I confirmed my name and date of birth, I climbed onto that wheeled cot and watched my mother huddle with Dr. Mickey again. Soon the Velcro from the wire across my forehead started to itch, and Dr. Mickey asked Dr. Larson, who was sitting on a stool with wheels, "Do you think Zofran could cause constipation? I just looked it up and think it's a definite possibility." Dr. Larson made a face indicating that while what Dr. Mickey was asking wasn't completely insane, it wasn't a question he'd been anticipating.

"How have you been feeling coming out of the anesthesia?" Dr. Larson asked, and it took me more than a few seconds to realize that I was now a part of this horribly intimate conversation about the state of my bowels.

"Oh . . . me?" I blurted. As I did a quick survey of the room, I noticed that more than one person was trying not to laugh at me. "Oh, so . . . I mean . . . other than a little drowsiness? I mean, that's really it. I know I'm never getting the year right and saying some stupid things, but the only side effect, really, is I'm just a little tired."

"Most people say very weird things when they're coming out of anesthesia, so don't worry about that. Are you ever nauseated? Do you ever feel like you want to throw up?"

"No, that's never happened," I answered. Dr. Larson asked me if I'd be willing to forgo the Zofran this time to see if it made any difference. I shrugged to indicate that I didn't see why not and then apologized for making them rearrange the medication for me yet again. They certainly didn't see me coming! One of only four percent of the population who hallucinates when given the tiniest dose of fentanyl and now I was constipated because of a small dose of anti-nausea medication.

Soon Dr. Larson was showing me the vials of propofol and lidocaine—the ritualistic, symbolic gesture of "We are about to do this to you, remember?"—and I gripped the blanket laid over me and found my mother's gaze across the room.

"If she talks your ear off while I'm out, I apologize," I announced without breaking eye contact with her. She slowly lifted her hand to flip me off. Yes, my devout Mormon mother flips me off routinely and once told me that because I love sex so much I should just find a stable man and get a gigolo on the side. I guess I hadn't realized just how much I had overshared until my Mormon mother used the word "gigolo."

"Dr. Mickey," I said, right before Dr. Larson set the lidocaine in motion, "my mother is flipping me off. This is what you have gotten yourself into."

His face instantly turned red and he laughed. "I love your mother's stories. She can talk all she wants."

I set my head back on the gurney and heard Dr. Larson say that he was beginning the propofol. Oddly, it burned going in this time. It hadn't ever burned, but I didn't care. I felt a line of fire sizzle up my arm into my shoulder. It didn't hurt, it just felt incredibly warm, and I thought the burning sensation might help my odds of outwitting the propofol. I began to say something about it; I opened my mouth and then . . . nothing.

I opened my eyes as they were wheeling me into the recovery room. I could feel the tiniest bit of a sticky residue on my left eye where they had taped it shut. They were so good to me, all of them—remembering the things that had made me uncomfortable or outright sick and adjusting their care to make it more pleasant. I didn't blurt out anything after waking up—which made me wonder if they were disappointed when they didn't get to go home and regale their friends and family with the crazy things that came out of our mouths when we were drunk on anesthesia.

I barely remembered the nurse's face, couldn't tell if I'd met him before, and when he asked me what year it was, I answered, "It's 1979."

Everyone in the room got really quiet again except for my step-father, who started laughing uncontrollably. I mean, it was objectively funny at this point. Why was I fixated on *that* year? Why not 1993, when I graduated from high school? Why not 1997, when I graduated from college? Why not, you know, the actual year?

The nurse asked, "Would you like to reconsider that answer?"

Listen, I love my kids and fight hard for human and animal rights, I always hold doors open for strangers, and I'm mostly a good person. But when he framed the question in that way, he flicked my drunk nerve and I answered, "Would you like to reconsider *your face*?"

Not my finest moment, I will admit this. Within a few seconds I realized it was 2017 and I felt so terrible. I apologized again and again and he kept reassuring me that he'd heard far worse things during his time doing this job.

We arrived home that afternoon, and for the first time since the treatments started I didn't want to be alone or rest or lie down in my bedroom. In fact, I felt an odd surge of energy I hadn't felt since before I'd begun training for the marathon.

My mother and stepfather offered to take my kids overnight to give me some time to reflect, maybe catch up on the work that was piling up, or just get some more rest. Since it was a Friday night, and because I had showered that morning and dressed in something I wouldn't wear to a Bikram Yoga class, I spontaneously drove over to a man's apartment, completely unannounced. He was a musician and the last person I'd met on Match.com before I canceled my subscription. Although I wasn't attracted to him, we talked about music and bands like we'd known each other for decades. He had played in bands that were popular in Provo, Utah, when I attended BYU. We knew several people in common, including a redheaded Mormon I'd dated who played guitar and reeked of sandalwood.

The musician didn't know I was sitting outside his apartment, so I texted him to let him know I was downstairs. This startled the hell out of him. Fifteen minutes later, he'd showered, cleared his living room floor of discarded socks and empty carry-out containers, unlocked his door, and let me inside. It was a total bachelor's apartment complete with a couch that looked like it had been dragged in from a curb near a train depot. His walls were covered haphazardly with concert posters. A dark blue sheet draped over the north-facing window was held in place by several thumbtacks. Two overturned buckets supported a plank of wood to make a coffee table. I felt like I had stepped into a tree house.

"I would have rolled out the red carpet if I'd known you were coming over," he mumbled as he gathered up more trash to hide in one of the kitchen cupboards. "Wanna have a seat?" He gestured toward the scavenged couch, which sat opposite a giant, makeshift stereo system complete with two record players.

"Yeah, sure," I said, and I patted the cushion to make sure it wasn't wet before I took my place.

"Can I get you a beer? I remember you said you didn't like beer, but I don't have any wine. Why didn't you tell me you were coming over so that I could prepare?"

"A beer is fine."

"I can't believe you're seeing my place in this condition," he said as he shoved several pairs of shoes into his bedroom.

"What condition is it usually in?" I said smirking.

"Funny. You think you're funny." We had this rapport, like two siblings who only communicate by ribbing each other. He brought me a beer from a tiny fridge, and after he handed it to me he turned toward the stereo system.

On the first and only date we'd been on, he had played me a mix

CD he'd made of early nineties music—literally a CD in a CD player mounted in his dashboard.

He was driving me home from dinner. We'd had sushi and drunk sake while reminiscing about life back in Provo, all the people we knew in common. How that sandalwood-reeking redhead who broke the honor code by piercing his ears and nose was now a straitlaced father of three and recently served as the bishop of his ward. And when one song faded into the next I heard the first note of a certain song and completely freaked out. It immediately transported me into my 1987 gray Honda Accord with a CD system I'd bought at Radio Shack. My stepfather had installed it before I left for college, before I made that thirty-two-hour nonstop drive from Memphis, Tennessee, to Provo, Utah. I impulsively gripped his arm while gasping for air.

"Wait . . . is this . . . OH MY GOD. This . . . this . . ." I was trying to place it, trying to put it all together in my head.

"You know this song?" he asked incredulously, and tried to keep his eyes on the road. "I have never been out with a woman who knows this song."

The lead singer finally came in with the opening lyric: "And then she smiled . . ."

It all finally came back to me. The CD I had played over and over again in my car on the drive back and forth between my house, the job I worked at a bakery, and the parking lot on campus. They were a British band called Adorable from the early nineties who put out a couple of albums, and the one I listened to, *Against Perfection*, was out of production. I'd tried many times to find it on iTunes and then on streaming services but only spotted it once on eBay for a ridiculous amount of money. When the song eventually got to the chorus—"Sunshine smile, sunshine smile"—I was belting the words right along with it like a ridiculous karaoke drunk. I hadn't heard that line in almost twenty years and it felt like my dog had gone missing and then someone showed up at my door with her safely cuddled in their arms. Total auditory elation.

Now he went to the stereo system and picked up a large square of cardboard covered with the image of a flower on fire. "You know I have the whole record, right?" He waved it at me.

"Wait . . . is that . . ." The image looked somewhat familiar.

"Adorable. Remember? You said you couldn't get your hands on a copy of it. I have the actual *record*."

"Oh my God—"

"That's right, oh my God."

"Please. Please will you play 'Homeboy'?"

He turned back toward the stereo system, pulled the black vinyl from its cover, and placed it on the turntable. After making adjustments on a few knobs, he placed the needle directly into the perfect groove. The song begins with a driving bassline backed by a minimal drumbeat that is unmistakable. I could smell the bread I used to pull out of the oven at that bakery back in 1996. Floods of memories of joking around with coworkers, walking through campus from one class to another, opening the window in the second-floor room I shared with a fellow English major named Amy, and admiring the blooms on the tree that reached up past the roof. I remember falling in love with Utah.

I couldn't move. I just sat there and let the memories wash over my body in one electrifying wave after another. When the lead singer got to the chorus—"You're so beautiful!"—the song exploded with crashing swells of guitar. I started to cry. I felt each chord in every molecule of my body and the back of my brain began to vibrate.

"Hey, you okay?" he asked, and walked over to sit next to me.

"Yeah. I'm good. Let me hear the whole song, okay?" I don't

know how I managed to get the words out of my mouth. My entire nervous system was quivering. By the end of the song the lead singer was yelling, "You're so beautiful!" and I'd eagerly anticipated it. Every hair on my body stood up from the chills all over my skin. When it ended, I continued to vibrate and cry.

"You sure you're okay?" he asked again.

I wiped the tears from my cheeks and nodded. "I can't remember the last time I heard a song that made me feel like that," I explained. "I mean, it used to happen all the time."

"It's a great song."

"It's not that," I continued. "It is an amazing song, but it's just that . . . that was . . . that was like hearing music for the first time. Like I'd been deaf and I finally heard a chord. I heard harmony."

"Dude, are you trippin'?" He was asking seriously. He didn't know that I had willingly let an anesthesiologist flatten my brain waves five times in the last ten days. He couldn't understand the significance of the sound of that song.

I had heard music. I had felt it. And while I had listened to that bassline and that chorus and that explosion of guitar before, its beauty was now magnified a million times over.

We played the rest of the album while chatting about his job, our friends, our common Southern upbringing. His mop of long hair was still wet from the very quick shower he'd taken while I sat in my car outside. It stuck out from underneath a wool hat he'd pulled down over his ears. In the afterglow of that song he looked cute, more attractive than I had found him on our first date. When we reached a natural pause, I told him I needed to head home. I was feeling a bit tired from the treatment and wanted to take full advantage of an empty house and the possibility of sleeping for an indulgent amount of time.

He walked me downstairs, past the entrance to the auto repair shop underneath his apartment, and out through the wire mesh gate to my car. When I opened my door, he reached out to touch my arm.

"When do I get to see you again?" he asked. His fingers brushed up against my elbow. I don't know what came over me or why I did what I did or who I was in that moment, but I stepped toward him and reached up to kiss him squarely on his mouth. I lingered there for a few purposeful seconds.

"Soon," I answered as I pulled away. His face was frozen in a stunned expression. I put my hand on his right cheek and stroked it.

He blinked several times and then put his hand on mine. "I told you that you were gonna like me! And I ain't ever wrong!"

I smiled and then climbed into my car. As I drove away we both waved, and I started to cry again. Tears slowly trickled out of my eyes. I let them puddle on my shirt and drove in silence the short distance to my house. When I pulled into my driveway, I turned off the ignition and peered at the porch light above me.

I didn't want to get ahead of myself. I didn't want to assign too much meaning to what had happened. I'd felt "Homeboy" enter my body and shake it awake. I'd laughed with him so easily about crazy Southern relatives who yelled things like "I'm hungry enough to straddle a dead pig and eat a bologna sandwich." And when I'd reached up to kiss him? *Kissing?*

I felt so alive. I wanted to breathe in this feeling. This buzzing hadn't stopped since the bassline of that song. And then I had a very specific thought:

Do I really *want to be dead?* Really?

FOURTEEN
MELTING SNOW

THE FOLLOWING DAY WAS a Saturday. I remember it so vividly because it was unseasonably warm. By early afternoon I was sitting out on my front porch, watching Leta and Marlo zip by on their scooters, up and down the small street that we'd moved to not three weeks before. This was the first time in their entire lives that we lived in a house on a flat side street, a street where they could finally live out the fullness of their childhoods and ride bikes and scooters in the street without battling a hill or worrying about getting plowed down by a minivan. We'd always lived on busy, hilly streets. One was so steep that a tractor snowblower once got away from my ex-husband and raced down the sidewalk into our neighbor's fence. We'd never met that neighbor, and so we pretended that nothing had happened.

Two months prior to the move, my therapist made me set two specific goals that she knew would help improve my mental health. One, I needed to move out of my ridiculously enormous house into the small and cozy home up for rent across town. Two, I needed to quit my job at the nonprofit. Both of these decisions terrified me. They paralyzed me. How could I possibly organize a move when I did not want to be alive? Does she not know that I have raised two packrats, one who will eat Hi-Chews and stash the wrappers in her closet just in case she ever needs them? And quitting the job? *Was she insane?* Yes, I hated the work, and seeing my boss's name gave me instant panic attacks, but at least it provided stability? I use a question mark because even though I collected a monthly paycheck, that job had thrown me into a hole so deep that even a good day would rank as unstable. These decisions involved talking to two people: my landlord and my boss. I was going to put a little bit of a dent into their normal routines. Did I mention that I hate conflict? Like, I do not like being a burden. My therapist had to force me to ask for help with my laundry, for God's sake. When I sense potential conflict, I'm like a turtle retreating into its shell. You can pick me up and shake me and my head will not ever poke out except to say, "Oh, did you just do something to hurt me? I'm so sorry! Here, take my wallet. Here are the keys to my house! Can I fix you a cup of coffee? Or would you prefer a back rub? We good? Good. Glad that's all cleared up!"

I made that call to my landlord. Then I wished I could get back all those hours I'd wasted worrying that it was going to be the most awful phone call of my life. I detected a sense of relief on the other end of the line when I told her that I was giving her thirty days' notice. I was renting a 5,800-square-foot house for a total steal yet drowning underneath the weight of the price of gas and electricity and snow removal and the ridiculousness of 5,800 square feet. In fact, to offset rent and utilities, I sublet two rooms in the basement. One was to an adorably odd lady in her sixties who often cooked eggs and salmon in my microwave. The house would reek with the stench of it, and often the girls would come home from school and start crying because Susan just had to have her fish. I'd had to tell Susan, too, that we were vacating the house. That was a terribly hard conversation to have until we reminisced about the night the basement flooded and we both had to pretend in front of my landlord that Walter, the older man renting the other room, was my fiancé.

A month after that phone call, my entire family and several of their Mormon comrades showed up to my house to move 5,800 square feet of stuff, including a mountain of Hi-Chew wrappers into a 1,300-square-foot space. Except it snowed over 18 inches during the night and we couldn't get the moving truck up the giant hill to the house. Which is one of the reasons that particular Saturday morning stuck out so vividly for me. The snow had melted and I'd hung pictures in the new living room. The move was over, many thanks to the Mormon Battalion, and I was . . . I felt . . . I was sitting on the porch with sunlight pouring down on my toes over the awning and I did not want to be dead.

Had I really wanted to be dead? Had I *really* felt that way? Because I didn't want to be dead anymore. Not at all. The sun was out and my beautiful kids were being kids. I was watching them live out their childhood in the street just beyond the lawn, zipping back and forth, their heads thrown back in laughter. My beautiful, tender girls. My flesh and blood. My life.

My phone was sitting in my lap, and suddenly as Marlo passed by on her scooter—she had oven mitts over her elbows and knees affixed with rubber bands because we hadn't bought proper safety gear yet—I remembered that Dr. Mickey had given me his card with his phone number on it. He'd handed it to me during our initial interview and told me to call him with any concerns, big or little. So I ran inside the house, found the card inside my wallet, and then ran back outside to enjoy the porch a little longer.

At 3:42 p.m. on March 18, 2017, I sent Dr. Brian Mickey the following text:

"Hey, Dr. Mickey. I hope you don't mind me texting you on your personal line. I just needed to tell you that I am experiencing a kind of hope and happiness today (and yesterday) that I thought wasn't possible again. It almost feels strange, like a limb I lost that suddenly reappeared. It feels . . . great."

Moments later, he responded:

"I don't mind . . . Is this Heather?"

"Yes. This is Heather."

"I thought so. So glad to hear you're doing well!"

"Thank you."

And that was it.

I had said it.

Well, I had texted it, but giving voice to those feelings felt . . . right. And I wanted him to be the first to know.

The first to know that it was working.

———

You want to know what else worked? Remember the woman who experienced constipation when administered Zofran? Yeah. She tried poop tea for a second time. Drank a cup of it that Saturday morning and by late afternoon found herself abruptly lying on the cold tiles of the bathroom floor, thinking she was going to die. She no longer *wanted* to be dead—she was now certain of this—but it turns out that when poop tea works, you can't undo it. She actually texted her mother from that bathroom floor: "UNDO POOP TEA. UNDO."

Her mother texted back, "Don't ever drink that tea if you have plans to be more than ten feet from a toilet."

FIFTEEN

IN THE NAME OF JESUS CHRIST, AMEN

THE DAY AFTER I texted Dr. Mickey was a Sunday. The weather was nothing short of brilliant. The clear blue sky stretched for miles and all the recent snow had melted, so I spent most of the day outside enjoying a two-day break from flatlining. Dr. Bushnell would eventually clarify that they weren't technically killing me; it was more of a really, really intense induced coma. They were just *almost* killing me.

During the early afternoon hours I was playing fetch with my miniature Australian shepherd, Coco. She was either born without a brain or, if she does biologically possess one, it operates in only three modes: cuddle, protect, or attack anything that comes close to her flock. That last mode is trigger-happy, and it has only gotten worse as she's aged. And as I mentioned previously, she also likes to scream and flip her body in the air when I let her out of her crate to feed her. She's ten years old and been solely in my care since the divorce.

I'm not sure why my ex-husband didn't show any interest in our (then) two dogs when I asked for the separation over six years ago. He didn't ever ask to walk them or spend time with them or fight for shared custody. He just sort of exited their lives. Our other dog, Chuck, was a mutt who took that absence a lot more personally than Coco. Chuck was a lovable Grinch who became famous on my website because I routinely posted pictures of him balancing odd objects on his head: cereal boxes, jars of peanut butter, beer bottles . . . When Jon left, Chuck's mood and health took a nosedive.

I really miss that little guy, and it was soon after his death in 2015 that I started training for the Boston Marathon. I just now put that together. I loved that dog so much and miss him terribly. I continue to find stray dominoes in the sequence that led to that gurney.

Coco doesn't have moods, she has a job. Moods are distracting and so is any moving object that comes within five hundred yards of her flock. That includes me and the girls, of course, but it expands when we are with family and friends to include all of them. She was put on this earth to protect us and scream deafening yelps of triumph when we walk through the door, because that means she did not lose us. She'd also rather play fetch than eat. This afternoon I was throwing a yellow lacrosse ball in the backyard. After seven years of research I finally determined that this is the only object she cannot destroy. My mother texted me and asked if I could talk. She had something on her mind that she needed to tell me.

Coco had just brought the ball back to me, and I picked it up and walked over to the steps leading out of the sliding door from Leta's room onto the back porch. As I sat down I called my mother and motioned for Coco to follow me and lie down.

"Hey," I said. "What's up? Everything okay?" Usually she just texts and says, "Can you talk?" But this text had said, "Can you talk? I have something important I need to ask you." I knew this wasn't going to be a regular checkup call about the girls or our plans for the day.

"Yeah, everything is fine. I just . . ." She breathed a sigh so heavy that I involuntarily stood up and began to pace slowly around the porch. "I want to ask you something, and I know it's a sensitive topic. But please hear me out."

"Of course," I assured her. She'd been, well, my angel these last two weeks, as gross as it is to write that; my angel.

"Your father . . . ," she began, and upon hearing that word I felt my body start to seize up. "I know we had talked about keeping this a secret from your father. Well, not necessarily a secret, but you know what I mean."

"We didn't want to hear his opinion," I said. "He just doesn't need to know."

"I know, he doesn't," she agreed. "Except, when he calls me and asks how I'm doing, I don't even know what to say to him. I mean, most of my recent life has been spent at that clinic."

"I know," I said, and started to feel a familiar sense of guilt.

"Heather, I know Rob is there with me when you go under, but I feel incredibly alone in all of this. The father of my baby girl has no idea what she has committed her body and mind to, what you are sacrificing. The father of my child isn't in there watching your eyes flutter shut and your body go limp and the staff struggling to get that breathing tube down your throat. I have no idea what to say to him, because everything is not just *fine*."

"I'm so sorry," I said.

"I don't think you know this but I don't sit down or stop feeling anxious or stop holding my own breath until the moment they take that tube out of your mouth and I see your chest moving up and down on its own. When I see you breathing again, it's almost more than I can take. The relief almost knocks me out."

"Mom, I am so sorry. You don't have to be in the room. I hate that I am doing this to you."

"You aren't doing anything to me. I told you, we were going to get through this together. And I am so proud of you for taking this leap, for making such a formidable decision. You are so brave to be doing this, and I am privileged to be in that room. I want to be there." Her voice was trembling. "I just woke up this morning and realized that watching you go through this has had such an effect on me. It's a heavy thing; it's a lot. But I am so happy to be in that room."

"*Of course* I want you in there. And if telling Dad about this will ease any of this burden, I will gladly call him." I laughed a bit at the thought of it. I'd be glad to call him and tell him that I had been dying every other day for the last ten days. Then, while he's still in shock, I may as well come clean about all the lesbian porn I masturbate to.

"You'd do that? For me?" my mother asked.

"I'd do that for you, Mom," I assured her. "I'll call him this afternoon."

"There's one other thing," she said. "Remember how we talked about your brother and sister coming and watching a treatment?"

I did remember. We'd tossed around that idea, since the depression and anxiety in our family has affected so many of the grandchildren—my nieces and nephews, my own children.

"Have you talked to them about it?" she asked. I hadn't. I'd been silent about it all because what if it didn't work? Then what?

Except . . . *I think it* had *worked*.

"Well, I have talked to them about it," she said, "and both of them said they could take off of work to come with us tomorrow."

"Tomorrow? Oh! That soon," I said surprised. "Yeah, that would be amazing if they could be there."

"Great. I'll call them and arrange everything. We'll probably all meet at your house and drive up together."

"Sounds good," I said. "I'll call Dad in just a minute. I need to take a few deep breaths and maybe a few shots of tequila before I do."

"Thank you," my mother whispered on the other end. "I am so proud of you."

"One more thing, Mom."

"What's that?" she asked.

"I feel good. I feel different. Very different."

"What do you mean?"

"Like, I feel like laughing and spinning in circles. I kind of want to just lie down in the grass under the sun and breathe in the feeling of being alive. Does that make sense?"

"Yes, it does," she said. "You know, I've been watching you this whole last week and it has felt like you were on the verge of something. There was more light in your eyes, less heaviness in your voice. And I didn't know if it was because you were starting to feel better or if it was just because you had hope."

"I definitely had hope," I explained. "But some switch got flipped on Friday. Something happened. Maybe that was the magical reset that Dr. Bushnell talked about. Or maybe it was the cumulative effect of all the treatments before it. I don't know, and I don't really care. Something happened. My life changed on Friday. I heard music again."

"Oh, Heather . . ." I could hear her voice verging on a cry. "I knew this would work. I know you don't believe in prayer, but I do." And then she was sobbing. "I knew the Lord would answer my prayers, the prayers of all of us who have been rooting for you. There are so many of us. And I truly believe that the Lord is the reason you were sitting in that doctor's office on that specific day. He led you there. I knew this would work."

My family and I have a mutual respect for our differing religious beliefs, theirs being in the Mormon faith, mine being in science. I've chosen to raise my girls without a specific religion: they both know that their father and I do not believe in a god, and yet both of them are polite and treat people with warmth and respect and they know right from wrong. They witness my extended family praying over meals and before bedtime and have attended church with them a few times, and I would have no issue at all if either of them decided to adopt the religion. It will have been their choice and theirs alone, a choice I felt like I had never been given. However, I don't think I made that clear enough to Leta, who one night at the age of eleven said she desperately needed to talk to me about something but was afraid that I was going to be furious with her. My mind immediately rushed to something she could have googled. After she got ready for bed, we sat side by side against her headboard as she summoned the courage to talk to me. I'm certain her heart was racing as fast as mine was, and she took several deep breaths before saying a word.

"You promise you won't be mad at me?" she finally blurted.

"Leta," I said, and instinctively reached out to stroke her head. "Remember what I told you? You can always come to me with any concern or worry or question, and no matter what it is, I will not get mad at you. I want you to have someone to talk to. I will always listen."

"I know. It's just . . . promise you won't be mad."

My heart started pounding even harder as the list of what she could possibly have done unspooled through my head.

"I believe in God!" she almost shouted.

I blinked hard, and I kept blinking for several more seconds without saying anything. *That* was what she was scared to tell me?

"I know you and Dad don't believe in God, but I do, and I have for a few months now."

"Oh, Leta." There was so much I wanted to say to her, but that was how I wanted to start: with her name.

"You promise you're not mad at me?" she pleaded, and she was dead serious.

"I am not mad at you," I promised her. "In fact, I am so happy that you told me."

"Really? *You're not mad?* But . . . I know you make fun of Mormons on your website, and—"

"I make fun of the fourteen-year-old Mormon that *I* was on my website. I wasn't a fun kid. The point is, I think it's wonderful that you believe in God."

"You do?"

"Yes! I always wanted you to make your own decision about it," I explained.

"Okay, but . . . there's more," she said.

"And what's that?"

"Sometimes I like to pray, too."

"You like to pray?"

"Yeah. Like, sometimes when I'm feeling anxious, it brings me comfort. It, like, calms me down."

"Leta, I think this is all wonderful. How amazing that you have found something you can do and connect to that brings you comfort."

"You're really not mad about that?"

"No! Not at all. In fact, I'd be willing to pray with you sometimes if you want me to. I was a pro at it back in the day."

"*You prayed?*" She could not believe these revelations.

"I did. I was a very good Mormon when I was a Mormon. I'll even take you to church if you want me to—"

"NO! I'm fine. I don't need to go to church. I just want to believe in God and pray."

I laughed with my whole body. Of all the reasons I left the church, that three-hour block of weekly boredom on Sunday mornings was very near the top.

I prayed with her that night and let her lead. She used some of the common language Mormons use in prayers, like "Please keep all of our loved ones safe" and "We thank You for our home and our health."

"In the name of Jesus Christ, amen."

The fact that my mother was convinced that the success of my treatment was all the Lord's doing did not bother me. How could it? She had sacrificed so much for me in the last ten days. If she thought that her Lord and Savior had put me in the right place at the right time, I was happy with her believing it and sharing that belief with me.

Also, a switch had flipped. That's the only way I can describe it. I was Dorothy opening the door of her house when it landed in Oz. The colors were nearly blinding.

———

About a half hour later, I had thrown that yellow lacrosse ball across the yard so many times I thought my arm might fall off. This dog would fetch a ball until she fell over, and even then she'd beg for you to throw it again. I let her in the side door of the house and walked to the front porch to sit in the afternoon sun.

It had worked.

I kept repeating the words in my head: *It worked. It worked.* I didn't want to be dead anymore. That was all that mattered. Whatever reaction my father had would be secondary to this fact.

I found his contact on my phone and dialed his number nervously.

"Feather! Is that you?" he asked. The story goes that he wanted to name me Heather so that at the end of the day when I was out in the neighborhood playing with friends and it was time to come home for dinner, he could step outside, cup his hands around his mouth, and yell, "Come hither, Heather Hamilton!" I remember that he did this a few times, but his nickname for me, Heather Feather, is the one thing about our relationship that hasn't ever really changed. He calls me that every time he speaks to me, and because he is my father and I am his daughter, it softens the edges of our many differences.

"Hey, Dad. It's me. How are you guys?" I said "you guys" because I knew he would put me on speakerphone and my stepmother would hear the entire conversation. I cannot remember the last time I spoke with my father when she was not listening. I don't have private conversations with my father, and I believe this dynamic has contributed to the distance between us.

"We're good! It's good to hear from you! How is everything?" I could hear my stepmother walking across the room in the background.

"The girls are great and we're slowly getting settled into the house. I've got a few photos hanging up in the living room. My office is a bit of a mess, but I'll get to that soon."

We continued for several minutes to make small talk about the weather and my stepbrothers and their families, and then I stood up to pace around the front lawn. When we got to a natural pause in the conversation, I just blurted it out.

"I have something to tell you, something really important. This is why I called."

"Okay," he said. If I know anything about my father I'm confident that he straightened his back to take in the news. "What's up, daughter of mine?"

"I'm telling you this at Mom's urging, mostly, because she's carrying a lot right now. And it doesn't feel right to make her carry it all."

"Okay. What is she carrying?"

"So, basically . . . I think you might have some idea about how depressed I've been over the last year or so, right?" I asked, expecting him to have no idea whatsoever.

"Well, now, I know your job has been hard on you. We've talked a bit about that. Is there more to it than your job?"

"Yeah, it's my job and all that training I did for the marathon and my diet and the ongoing, relentless pace of taking care of two kids alone. I haven't had a very good year."

"I didn't realize it was that bad, darlin'." He's lived in Utah for over a decade and yet, like every other person in my family, he hadn't been able to shake the Southern drawl.

"It's bad. Like, really, *really* bad. Or at least it was. It was the worst episode of depression I've ever experienced. Mom was probably the only one who knew the extent of it."

"Well, I'm sorry to hear that. Is there something we can do for you?" he asked.

"So, hm . . . how do I put this . . . I think what I need from you right now is to let Mom talk to you about what she's been witnessing. She feels alone because she and Rob have been taking me up to the ECT clinic for the last ten days or so to go through an experimental treatment."

"ECT?" he asked gravely. "You mean *electroshock therapy*?"

"I'm not getting electroshock therapy, Dad. No. This treatment is being conducted at the same clinic is all."

"Oh, wow. Wow. Okay, so tell me about it."

I laid it all out in very basic terms. I used harmless language so as not to alarm him any more than he already was. But when I finally got to the part about the breathing tube, I found myself becoming firm.

"I don't know what happens when I am out. I have no clue. I'm awake and then suddenly I'm in another room waking up from the anesthesia, saying crazy things and sometimes berating strangers. I have no idea what goes on when I'm under. But Mom is in there the whole time watching this happen, and some of it is unsettling for her. Some of it is *devastating*, even. But I will let her tell you about it. I mean, I have no idea what she's seeing. I just know that this has been really hard on her."

My stepmother piped up in the background. "What made you decide that this was safe? I mean, how many people have done this?"

"I am only the third participant. Two have gone before me, and according to my doctor both of them reacted well to the treatment."

"But what made *you* decide?" she persisted.

"Like I said, I was really, really depressed. I guess I thought that nothing was going help. I didn't think I would ever be able to climb out of it; that's what scared me most. I once told Mom that it felt like the nervous breakdown from which I would never recover. The idea of this treatment was far less scary than thinking I was going to feel like that for the rest of my life. Plus, I trust my doctor. He's the smartest man I know and has revolutionized ECT. He assured me that I'd be safe."

There was a long, uncomfortable pause in the conversation.

"My kids deserve to have a happy mom," I added. "I know it may seem to you like it's too big of a risk in terms of them, but I chose to do it *for them*."

"Well, do you think it's gonna work?" she asked.

At the risk of sounding unnecessarily harsh and completely unfair, I didn't think that they deserved to know just yet. They hadn't been in that room. They hadn't driven me up the winding streets to the clinic and sat with me as I filled out forms and battled 22-gauge needles. They had not witnessed what my mother witnessed when my brain would go down so hard and so fast that the assembled crew had to struggle with my limp body. They had never battled lingering, incapacitating feelings of sadness and not understanding that sadness, just knowing that they wanted that sadness to end.

"I'm hopeful," I said.

"Well, okay. If you say so!" she said, and chuckled.

"Feather, thanks for telling us all this. It's a lot," my father said, taking back control of the conversation. "I'll talk to your mother, probably today or tomorrow."

He would call my mother that evening and listen to her describe the last ten days of her life, perhaps the most harrowing she'd lived through in recent memory. He didn't offer much insight—how could he?—and told her that he was sorry she felt like she was going through this alone. I don't think my father remembers cornering me in my room or yelling at my brother or any of the comments he made about a woman's body in front of me or my sister. I don't think he knows just how much my fear of his temper shaped my life. I used to think that our relationship would transform when I had my own kids because my dad loves babies, but that didn't ever really happen. He doesn't spend much time with my girls, and while my girls don't mind spending time with him, they just don't see him very often. Most of what we share revolves around practical things he knows about and can advise me on, like financial planning and relationships with employees and bosses and where to do research when I'm shopping for a major purchase.

This has always been somewhat fine with me, our dynamic, our relationship. After my parents divorced, he moved several miles down the road and I lived with my mother 100 percent of the time. She was the one who influenced my transformative years, and so a father figure to me is someone who shows up to a volleyball game and a choir concert and occasionally dispenses advice on how to save money and open a checking account. I love him dearly—I have always loved him dearly—and I do have fond memories of him from my childhood that mostly include the hysterical way he could imitate Donald Duck. I remember riding on his shoulders as we walked through the neighborhood so that I could reach up and touch the leaves of trees. I remember when he would dress me for church in a T-shirt printed to look like a prison uniform to make my mom laugh. He taught me to be kind to strangers and smile at every person working the checkout line at the grocery store and why a good credit score is important. He truly has given me so much.

But, sadly, he is not someone I would ever call if I were in a crisis. I would not think to dial his number if I got a flat tire on the freeway and had run out of options. In fact, the day before we moved houses, before I had started treatment, I dropped the girls off at piano lessons and then ran back home to load up the car. There were some things I wanted to move into the house myself, things I didn't want misplaced or mishandled by a team of movers who would not understand their value. After packing the back seats full, I climbed into the driver's seat to turn on the car and race back to pick up the girls, but my car would not start. That house sat across town from the piano teacher's home, and there I was, stuck in a hybrid vehicle with an engine that wouldn't turn over. I had no idea what I was going to do. I called my mother and did what I had been doing for over nine months: I started screaming, which always goes over well and fixes everything.

I was totally shaken, tired, exhausted—all of it. I had no one to pick up my kids, didn't know how I was going to get them to school in the morning, didn't know how I was going to get the car where it needed to go to get fixed. My mother attempted to calm me down and offered to drive over and pick up the girls. Suddenly a very specific and lonely feeling overcame me.

"WHERE IS MY FATHER! WHERE IS MY DAD!"

I was not asking questions. I was screaming declarations. The words shook the car.

"WHY IS HE NOT HERE! WHERE IS MY FATHER!"

I yelled this over and over, and my mother did not stop me. She just listened. When I finally stopped, she asked where I was.

"I'm sitting in the car that will not start."

"Stay in the car and give me five minutes, okay? Five minutes. Just breathe. Can you do that? Do this for me. I will call you back in five minutes."

I agreed and sat in that driver's seat slouched over the steering wheel, sobbing. My God, how much crying had I done? I felt so stupid and helpless and more than anything completely hopeless. Hopelessness consumed me, paralyzed me, rendered me useless. Everyone would be better off without me.

Less than three minutes later my mother called me back.

"Your father is leaving his house right now. He'll be there as soon as he can, probably in less than a half hour. He is going to help you with your car."

"But I don't—"

"You don't anything. Your father is coming. Period. End of discussion."

"What did you tell him?"

"You don't want to know what I said to that man." I could hear her anger.

"About me?" I didn't want my father to know how hysterical I was.

"Not about you, no," my mother assured me. "I said what I needed to say, I'll put it that way. He will be there soon. Hang on until he gets there."

Twenty minutes later he and my stepmother pulled into my driveway. I have no idea how they got there so fast, given how far away they live and my father's unwillingness to break any laws, ever. I'd had very little time to fix my face after crying. My mother must have said what she needed to say.

We tried to jump the car with cables, but we failed over and over again. We assumed that because it was a hybrid, something could be wrong with any of the eleven computers inside the car's system. Together we made a list of places to call, and I sat with my stepmother in my living room as my father called every place on that list to get a quote on a new battery, making sure he could find the cheapest one available. If it wasn't the battery, we'd take it to the dealership and have them assess the problem.

He'd shown up. My dad had finally shown up, and maybe that's because I had finally given him the chance to show up. My God, what I would give to know what my mother said to him. She refused to tell me, except that she'd scared the living shit out of him. So I am just going to assume that it had to do with his pension and reminding him that she hadn't asked for a single dime of it in their divorce.

I did not know that my mother was taking notes during each treatment and keeping a journal of our time spent together. I had been jotting down notes of my own but had no idea she was doing the same. The day before she asked me to call my father she wrote the following entry in her notebook:

Mom's Personal Journal Page
March 18th, 2017

Three treatments this week. Such a long week!! So emotionally draining. I am sure it is physically stressful but I have not allowed myself to stop and realize that feeling for months. My body has been on high alert in case Heather needs my and Rob's help. However, I realized today that we are at the halfway point of these treatments and I can no longer carry this burden without the help of her father. Even though we have been divorced for over 30 years, our role and bond as parents have never ceased. She was our last child and his love for his "Feather" is tender even though he sometimes doesn't get her!!

Heather has chosen not to let him know about the treatments. I have had frequent conversations with him and her stepmother during this time and I constantly have had to skirt the fact that we are spending so much time watching her slip into the abyss. They haven't a clue what is happening. How would I tell them about the first treatment and have them fully understand my fear as I watched them hook her up to all the monitors and start the anesthetic. I doubt anyone could fully comprehend my dread as I saw the fear in her eyes a second before she went under. I watched at the foot of her bed as they shoved the breathing tube into her throat and started the oxygen to keep her alive. I followed all the machines as the doctors explained their functions. But I mostly watched her artificial breaths register as she literally slipped into the deepest abyss possible for the brain, zero. I did not exhale for sometimes 30 minutes until they could remove the tube and her own breathing began to register on the monitor, irregularly at first but then smooth, beautiful breaths!! Trust me! The Lord knew all about all of this because I told him about every tiny part of it as I begged him to keep her safe and heal her over and over again. I think he finally said ENOUGH! I HAVE THIS! SHE WILL MAKE IT THROUGH THIS!!

Her brother and sister knew and I shared every detail with them. Now her father needed to know and share the process. I wasn't sure how Heather would react to this request.

SIXTEEN

ON BEHALF OF LOVED ONES LONG PASSED

LATE MONDAY MORNING MY brother and sister both showed up at my new place before my sixth treatment. We'd seen more of each other in the last two weeks than we had the entire year. There is a part of me that wishes we were all closer to each other than we are, but I know how unrealistic that wish is. Both of my siblings have five kids, which means they have to manage five different, ridiculous schedules. They and their spouses both work, and when you take a look at my schedule and how angry I get when someone has the gall to call me during my constantly thwarted attempts to complete All the Things Needing to Get Done, I think we are as close as we can possibly be. We wish each other happy birthday and gather for holidays and special events. We will text each other when our mom informs us that one of us is having a hard time.

But our shared heritage bonded us in a way that I am not bonded to anyone else. Our shared survival of the divorce and our continuing agony over certain things we endured during childhood make us feel a bit like we fought in a war together. Don't get me wrong: I know that our childhood was privileged and it could have been far worse than the relative luxury with which we grew up. But the three of us were in that trench together. We all grew up terrified of our father's temper.

All five of us climbed into the minivan and made the winding trip up to Colorow Way. My mother talked the entire time about the treatment, what they would see, who they would meet. I rolled up my sleeves to show them both my bruises, and my brother let out a "Holy crap!" He's by far the most left-leaning member of my family other than me, if "a centimeter to the left of right-wing" qualifies as left-leaning. But he is still a devout, practicing, Diet Coke–drinking Mormon who does not engage in profanity.

The bruises had spread several inches up and down my arms and they'd turned a gut-churning shade of brown. They didn't hurt as bad as they looked, but I wouldn't walk around in public without having them covered up.

I felt a little awkward walking in with my crew, all five of us, all *Southern* five of us. Each time we saw someone as we walked from the door to the waiting room, I said, "Hi! I decided to bring the entire state of Tennessee with me today. Hope you don't mind. They're polite and can make a mean bowl of cheese grits."

I walked up and said, "Yo!" to Greg, who winked while nodding at me. He had already printed out my wristband. After I signed in, he wrapped the wristband around my arm and handed me the clipboard with the sheet I always had to fill out. You know, the How Unbearable Is Life? one. I carried it back to a seat next to my mother, who was supervising my family, keeping them in line.

I printed my name at the top, filled in the date, and, without thinking, just glanced down at the questions. Falling asleep? Still no problem there. Sleeping during the night? Hm. I don't remember waking up during the night over the weekend. In fact, I'd slept really well. Feeling sad?

Wait.

Hold up.

I squinted as I tried to remember what I had checked before the fifth treatment. And then it hit me: I had checked the box next to "I feel sad nearly all of the time." Had I really checked that? *Really?* Had I felt like that? Why was I feeling that way? I literally had to squint to remember what it was like to feel that way. Because I wasn't sad. I hadn't felt sadness since . . . was it really *that* recently? I couldn't comprehend this sheet of paper. Without checking any boxes next to any of the questions on the front side of the paper, I flipped it over almost as if I'd stumbled on an ancient artifact.

The room almost started spinning, but not because anything was wrong. I just could not wrap my head around the rest of that sheet of paper.

11. View of Myself

On Friday I had checked the box next to "I think almost constantly about major and minor defects in myself." Three days ago. I had checked that. I believed that? I did? Why would I ever believe such a thing?

12. Thoughts of Death or Suicide

Suicide, of course, had never really been in the cards. But had I really felt that life was empty or wonder if it was worth living? I was now so happy to be alive that, without even realizing it, I had taken a shower and blown my hair dry that morning. I was starving the whole time, sure, but I'd put on clean clothes, worn a necklace, and even put on a dab of perfume. I hadn't considered how strange it was for me to have done those things without even thinking.

As I mentioned, there's this phenomenon with people who suffer from depression: often we can't really tell that we're feeling better after a change in medication or some other kind of help. It's usually the people around us who notice and have to point it out (like my roommates in college mentioning that I'd stopped slamming doors after I started taking Zoloft).

I would have eventually realized that I felt better when I went back to the psychiatrist for a follow-up visit and he asked me how I was feeling. When we're sad, we may express that we are sad, but the feeling is so overpowering that we aren't thinking about it as much as we are feeling it, enduring it. So when that feeling turns into happiness, it's just what we're feeling. Putting words to it whether by telling us about the difference or pulling those words out of us makes us realize the difference and appreciate it.

I knew that I didn't want to be dead anymore. I had seen color and heard music and wanted to breathe air. But I did not understand the significance of the change until I read the words on this piece of paper. It was life-changing.

13. General Interest

There was not an option that read "I am finally interested in music and books and television and movies and politics and writing stories about my kids and spending time with friends and walking my dog." I still hadn't had sex, but just sitting there, thinking about all the things I didn't even realize that I had missed so dearly, I suddenly thought, "A passionate kiss with tongue doesn't sound bad right about now. And wouldn't it be nice if someone touched my boob?"

I'd been checking the box next to "I have virtually no interest in formerly pursued activities" this whole time. I had the urge right then to run out of the clinic, drive straight to the airport, and hop a flight to New York, where I'd spend days doing nothing but walking around, taking photos, and listening to music. Other than my kids, there is nothing in life I love as much as walking around a city and taking photos while listening to music. Out of nowhere I blurted, "I haven't picked up my DSLR in over a year. A year!"

"Your what?" my mother asked, confused.

"My big camera. The one I used to pack with me on every trip. I used it every day for almost seven years and I haven't picked it up in over twelve months."

"Where did that realization come from?"

"This piece of paper, Mom. It's a revelation. I'm so glad they've made me fill it out, because do you understand what has happened here?"

"I have an idea," she said with a sly smile.

"No, I don't think anyone realizes what has happened here. The difference in how I feel now from what I felt just three days ago. How could . . . how could anyone possibly know?"

"You can see it in your eyes. If you hadn't said anything to me yesterday, I would have been able to tell by looking at you this morning."

"Really?"

"Well, first, your hair looks amazing and you smell incredible."

"Yeah, you know, I didn't even plan to shower this morning, I just did it. *Like a normal person.* I didn't even think about it."

"But your eyes are saying everything I need to know. They are beaming, and I can tell that the light inside them is coming from inside you."

As she said those words I could feel the light inside of me. I felt full of light. It was swelling inside my lungs.

Just then Lauren walked into the waiting room and approached me with her head cocked and a giant smile on her face. The ends of her hair were died a vibrant purple today.

"You look amazing!" she exclaimed while touching my shoulder. "I love this shirt. Where did you get it?"

I looked down at my shirt, having forgotten what I'd chosen that morning from my closet. It's so stuffed with shirts that if you aren't careful when you open it they all might topple onto your head.

"Oh, this thing?" I answered. "I subscribe to one of those services that sends me clothes, because if I had one wish in life it would be 'Please don't make me shop for anything at all whatsoever.'"

"Well, you look great today. Not that you haven't looked great every time you've been here, but today: Wow. And also, I'm saying that because I mean it, not because I'm buttering you up for the test you have to take."

"OH GOD, THE TEST!" I shouted. "Does everyone who takes this test get as nervous as I do? If they don't, please lie to me and tell me they do."

One of the things I agreed to when I signed up for this treatment was something that I did not want to agree to at all, not one bit. Yes, you can administer a dose of anesthesia that will make my brain nearly flatline, and fine, my mom can watch as you shake my body like a rag doll trying to get a breathing tube down my throat before I suffocate. But I am very hesitant to sign the waiver that states "may result in death" if you're gonna make me take a test afterward.

Before starting treatment, after the fifth treatment, and after finishing treatment, I would need to take what's called the Montreal Cognitive Assessment mental test. You may have heard of this test, as it is the test a physician gave to Donald Trump, who bragged that he had passed it with flying colors, and good for him. He can recognize the outline of a lion! Superior cognition.

Before this sixth treatment, Dr. Mickey called me back into an office to take the assessment test. But not before I'd joked with Lauren about how I wanted to throw up due to anxiety about it.

"I feel like I need to ace this test—like you guys are legally obligated to commit me if I don't."

"Don't sweat it. Today is Monday and we only commit people on Tuesdays."

Dr. Mickey sat across a desk from me in a windowless room next to Dr. Bushnell's office. "How are you feeling today, after the weekend?" he asked, holding a few sheets of paper in his hands.

"Right now I'd like to vomit," I answered. Then I realized that Dr. Mickey is not really familiar or comfortable with my style of humor. "Not because of you! It's just I hate tests. And you're making me take one. You're holding it in your hands. I see it. Right there. So I suppose technically it is because of you. But at some point I will forgive you, maybe. Overall I'm feeling really good! And I can't believe I just said that. With an exclamation point at the end, even."

"So you're still feeling like you did when you texted me on Saturday? And, yeah, sorry about the test. I'm sure you'll do fine."

"I *am* feeling just like I did when I texted you, yes," I assured him. "I feel like I can see color again. It's strange. I . . . I don't know what happened."

"This is great to hear. Great to hear," he said. I could tell that he might be thinking about the initial talk we had had before treatment began. He'd had to assess whether or not I was a good fit for the study, Dr. Bushnell's recommendation notwithstanding. I barely spoke during that interview, barely looked at him as he asked me several probing questions in the gentlest way. Did I think I was a good person? Did I think I was a worthy person? Did I have bad days or did I feel bad about life as a whole? It was when he asked about my kids that I totally lost it. I cried so hard that I had to wipe my face on my coat. He asked if I thought I was a good mother. Even though I knew I was taking care of all of their basic needs—food, laundry, school, piano, bedtime, etc.—I truly believed that they would be better off without me. I knew that they could sense my sadness. How could they not?

"So, the test . . ." He set down one of the pieces of paper. "I know you hate tests. But, again, let's take our time. There is no pressure here. You're going to do fine."

Telling someone with test anxiety not to have anxiety about a test is like telling an insecure thirteen-year-old girl that she shouldn't care what that cute boy in her science class thinks about her. She will care and she will obsess and she will fill entire diaries about it. I have the diaries to prove it.

"Before we do the written part of this, I am going to read you five words. And later on during the test I'm going to have you repeat them back to me in the same order, okay?"

I used to cram for exams in college and memorize answers only to forget them immediately after the exam. Like, *minutes* after. I ruined my memory by doing this so frequently that if you tell me your name and I don't make some complicated mental diagram of the letters in your name and a contorted association between your face and your name—"Jessica looks like she might be old enough to have watched *Happy Days* starring Ron Howard whose daughter

Bryce Dallas Howard has red hair, and Bryce Dallas Howard always reminds me of Jessica Chastain, so PHEW!"—I won't remember your face or who you are or how we met. Sorry!

I nodded and then tried to concentrate as hard as I could.

"Truck. Banana. Violin. Desk. Green." He said each word very deliberately and slowly. The first time I took the test I couldn't remember the word "daisy" even though that was my grandmother's name and I had considered naming a child after her. Thanks, Professors.

I repeated the words in my head and tried to draw some associations among all of them, when Dr. Mickey interrupted my meditation to move the test along.

"Okay, next. You see the numbers and letters here?" He pointed to the paper sitting in front of me. "Draw a line going from 1. to A and then from A to 2. and then from 2. to B, and so on, the numbers and alphabet being consecutive."

I didn't have a hard time with this part and finished by drawing a line from 5. to E. I breezed through it as if I could actually count. Me, the valedictorian! Who knew?

For the second part I had to draw a 3-D cube next to one printed on the paper, and it had to resemble the printed cube exactly. I used to draw cubes on the edges of my notebook in high school classes whenever I got bored, so this part did not faze me in the least. However, I knew I shouldn't get too cocky.

Because the next part, oh God. I was supposed to draw a clock with all of the numbers in the correct order and in the correct place on the clock, and I had to draw it to indicate that it was ten minutes past eleven o'clock. Meaning, I had to get the big and the little hands right, too. I had to think a lot harder than I should have about where the larger hand should go and in what direction, and because I've neglected my penmanship through years of typing and photo editing and texting, all the numbers were illegible. When I finished and admired my work, I set down my pencil and said, "I'm sure you've seen people take shits that look more like the face of a clock than that, and I apologize for being compelled to say this to you."

He laughed and waved it off like he always did when I said something inappropriate. Then we got to the fun part: identifying three animals based on detailed, very accurate outlines. First he pointed to the illustration of a giraffe and asked if I could tell him what it was.

"Is this part of the test for real?" I asked him.

He chuckled. "Yes, we're just making sure you can recognize basic things."

"That is, of course, a giraffe. I've seen one up close on a safari in Tanzania, which you definitely wanted to know about me. Ran a half marathon around the base of Mount Kilimanjaro. I'll stop talking now."

He smiled as he pointed to a bear.

"That would be a bear. Interesting story, my seventh grader has a teacher whose last name is Barriger, and when she introduced herself to the class she said, 'It's pronounced like a bear that goes, GRRR! Bear-ih-grrrrrr!' How am I doing? Am I identifying basic things?"

"You're doing great," he said as he pointed to the outline of a hippo.

"That would be a hippopotamus and I could regale you with story after story about how many people have sent me hippo-related paraphernalia over the years because I once wrote about this show I saw on *National Geographic* about a family in South Africa who adopted a hippo named Jessica and she slept in their house and the woman would give her nightly massages. And I realized that all I ever wanted in life was a pet hippo who would routinely break her bed. But I digress, Dr. Mickey."

Turns out being happy can make one quite talkative.

"Okay, I'm going to read you five numbers and I want you to say them back to me in the order that I read them. Ready?"

"Oh God. Fine."

He nodded and slowly read off of the sheet in his hands, "Two. Four. Eight. Five. Three."

I took a deep breath. "Two. Four. Eight. Five. Three."

"Okay," he said with no emotion. "Now I'm going to read you three numbers and I want you to say them to me in reverse order."

"You're killing me. I hate this part."

"Five. Two. Seven," he said slowly.

"Seven. Two. Five. Like, 'It's seven to five in the morning! He's supposed to be up cooking breakfast or something!'" He did not get the reference and I didn't think he would and if you don't, that's okay. A video went viral many years ago from a news segment in Oakland about people who were modifying the mufflers on their cars with whistle attachments, and other cranky people were complaining to the police about it. Someone they interviewed pointed out that all those grouchy people who heard the muffler sound in the early hours of the morning should already be awake and fixing their families breakfast. I have used that sentence at least once a day since I saw it when anyone complains about anything. You paid $200 for a haircut you hate? You're supposed to be up cooking breakfast or something!

The next part of the test had rattled me the first time I took it, because (1) I have no sense of rhythm, and (2) I startle easily. He was going to read me a list of letters, probably thirty in a row, and I would have to tap the desk each time he read aloud the letter *a*. When I first took this test, I kept jumping the gun whenever he read aloud an *f* because the beginning sounds like the letter *a*. At one point when I did tap the desk when he read aloud *f*, I'd shouted "I TAKE IT BACK!" Turns out you can't take back a mistake on a cognitive test.

This time he only read aloud three *f*'s in the long string of letters, and I'm pretty sure I aced that part, too.

Next he read two sentences to me and I had to repeat them back to him exactly as he'd read them. I don't remember what those sentences were, but I know I got them right because he smiled, nodded, and didn't make any notes. Even though I wanted to waste everyone's time by doing a victory dance, he moved immediately to the next part.

And then, oh God, one of the worst parts of this test—and, you guys, I graduated with a degree in English and make a living as a writer: I had one minute to name as many words as I could think of that began with the letter *f*. Surprisingly, I just didn't sit there and repeat the most obvious one over and over again, although I was tempted.

I reminded myself that the best way to get out as many words as possible was to go through all the vowels: words that begin with *fa*, words that begin with *fe*, words that begin with *fi*, and so on. I cannot recount how many words I got out in one minute or what each one was, but I do remember that *fart* was the first word I said. It begins with *fa*!

Dr. Mickey then asked me to describe the similarity between a train and a bicycle.

"They are both modes of transportation?" I asked.

He didn't hesitate. "Okay, what about the similarity between a ruler and a watch?"

"They are both used to measure things?"

"Good," he said, and I relaxed in my chair. Then he told me about the next part of the test. "Now it's time recall the words I read to you at the beginning of this. Can you tell me what those words are?"

I think the sweat from my armpits had soaked through the shirt Lauren had admired not even twenty minutes earlier. I'd made a mental image of each word in my brain in the seconds that Dr. Mickey had given me after reading those words to me.

"Okay, let's see . . . ," I said, hoping to impress him with basic mental skills. "Truck . . . um . . . banana . . . violin . . . desk . . . and . . . um . . . um . . . GREEN! GREEN! I got it! I know it's green because I sat at a green desk in seventh grade next to my friend who played the violin—I played the clarinet which wasn't nearly as prestigious, though I've gotten over that, maybe, but will I ever be as accomplished as she is?—and I know my favorite dessert in seventh grade was banana pudding, and since I grew up in the South, I am somewhat familiar with pickup trucks. *Phew.*"

Turns out being happy can turn one into one's super-talkative Mormon mother.

In those moments, Dr. Mickey always accommodated me with a smile, and I will be forever grateful for that generosity. That and the whole saving-my-life thing.

The last part asked me about my physical location—place, city, state—and about the day, month, year, and day of the week. Because I was not coming out of anesthesia, I easily nailed the year. Usually, I refer to my phone or watch to see what day of the month it is. I was really nervous, because I took a few seconds too long to come up with the right answer, and the only reason I got it right was because I counted forward three days from St. Patrick's Day, the day the switch had flipped.

I'll always have that association: the day of luck being one of the luckiest days of my life.

I was about to regale Dr. Mickey with a long explanation for why I have a hard time remembering dates but figured I had put him through enough. He then gathered my paper, placed it over his, and straightened them up.

"Like I said, I knew you'd do well," he said, stood up, and then motioned to the door. That's when I remembered, *Shit, my crew, the entire state of Tennessee, is waiting for me.* I hate making people wait for anything, and here I'd made them wait an extra twenty minutes while I drafted complex associations between bananas, violins, and trucks in my head so as to impress the doctor in charge of killing me.

Just as we made it back to the waiting room, a nurse said that they were ready for me. I looked over at my mother first, and she nodded at my brother and sister, who stood up slowly. We all entered the room with my gurney sitting at the opposite side, a flurry of activity going on around it. I confirmed my name and birthday as I walked toward the gurney, and before I could ask for a warm blanket, a nurse was offering me one. She handed it to me as I sat on that thin, crinkly mattress, and suddenly I had a terrible thought enter my head that I didn't have much time to process. It hit me so unexpectedly and with such force that I asked Dr. Mickey if he wouldn't mind coming closer so that I could ask him about it. He nodded and walked toward me while my mother arranged my crew around the walls of the room across from me.

"Could . . . could this treatment possibly reverse the effects of what happened last time?" I whispered when he was mostly out of earshot of everyone else. "I don't want to go back to life before last Friday."

His response startled me. He smiled more widely than I'd ever seen him smile, and Dr. Mickey is as boyish as a shy kid who is routinely given giant lollipops.

"No, I'm certain that it will not," he promised me. "In fact, the way this works, or is supposed to work . . . what we're replicating is a process wherein you only get better with each subsequent treatment. That is, if there is *any room* to get better. Since ECT usually involves ten to twelve rounds of treatment, we're trying to show that we can accomplish the same thing with fewer side effects. That's why each participant is doing ten. I'd never recommend you do another treatment if I didn't think it was only going to add to what you're experiencing."

I nodded as a nurse reached over and asked if I would lie back so that she could affix the Velcro wire to my forehead. I saw my mother pointing at me, most likely explaining everything to my brother and sister. Dr. Tadler was on call that day—thank God for Dr. Tadler. His presence was so comforting, maybe because he was considered the lead anesthesiologist for the study, or maybe because he had touched my arm like a concerned father before I entered the abyss for the first time. The anesthesiologist on call each day was written on a whiteboard outside of the waiting room, and we hoped to see his name every time we came to the clinic. When we did, my mother would do a move wherein she silently pumped both of her fists into the air followed by an awkward thumbs-up. God, I love her so much.

You tend to remember weird details about things when you're going under anesthesia. That time I remember looking up and not being drawn to my mother's eyes. I had found my sister's face, her beautifully angled and tan face. Her skin tone is so different from the blindingly pale tone of my own that some people have asked if we have the same parents, and so I introduce her as my half-Mexican sister. Her countenance was so heavy and burdened. That was the specific detail I remembered before . . . nothing. The nothingness. That deep and dark state of nothing. The abyss.

When I woke up, I blinked. On a few of my eyelashes I could

feel the remains of the tape they'd used to keep my eyes shut. My brother's face came slowly into focus. I don't remember if I said anything outrageously drunk, only that my brother saw that my eyes were focused on him. He immediately sat up straight in his chair and looked back at me sternly. And yet, it wasn't unfriendly or punishing. It was a signal for me to take him seriously.

"That was incredible," he said. "I don't know how to put into words what just happened in there. Just . . . incredible." He shook his head a little.

"Hey there," I heard a familiar voice to my right side. It was Chris, and it was good to recognize someone in that final room of all the rooms I had to walk through to get to the other side.

"Hey, Chris!" I said. "My name is Heather B. Armstrong! Beat you to it!"

"Excellent!" He was most likely being enthusiastic to amuse me. "Can you tell me what year it is?"

"It's 2012," I answered.

My stepfather started to laugh, and my brother let out a chuckle. I suppose my mother had prepped him for my stellar skill at getting the year wrong each and every time I came out of anesthesia.

"Why are you laughing?" I asked with drunk conviction. "Why is the fact that it's 2012 so funny? I don't get it."

"Are you sure it's 2012?" Chris asked.

I blinked a few more times and could feel the weight of the sticky eyelashes on my right eye hitting my lid. 2012, I thought; 2012. And then, as if someone were pulling me out of that year like a bucket out of a well, the years 2013, 2014, 2015, 2016, and finally 2017 appeared.

"Why do I do this every time? It's 2017. Sorry about that." And I always did feel sorry, like I was making their job harder to do. As a patient I only had one job to do. Well, really, only two jobs: one, die; two, wake up and get the date right. Why had they not fired me already?

Someone brought me a cup of apple juice without my even asking; I would later learn that my mother had gone around to each person working on the treatment to make sure that all the things I liked and needed were prepped and ready to go (including the warm blanket earlier). When I found my sister standing near my mother, I could see that her face was a little red, a warmer tint than her normal tan. I was a little too out of it to ask why, and I barely remember getting into the car and traveling the winding roads home—only that I hugged both siblings before they left and I climbed into my bed for an hour-long nap. Turns out that a weekend of feeling pretty happy about life is *exhausting*.

When I woke up, my mother and stepfather were in my living room waiting for me. The girls were at the library with the babysitter. I was awake enough, aware enough, to realize that I hadn't really gauged the reactions from my siblings. What had they really thought about it? Did they think I was insane? Did they think this was some sort of quackery?

"Just the opposite," my mother informed me.

"What do you mean?"

"Your sister, Heather. Your *sister*. As they were hooking you up to everything, I explained what was going on, how they all work together like this little machine to get you set up."

"I remember you pointing at me and talking to them."

"Well, Dr. Tadler held up the propofol and said he was ready to start. Do you remember that?"

Oddly, I hadn't remembered that part, and I usually did. I only remember looking up and seeing September's face, her concern and her worry.

"She saw your arms fall to your sides as you went under and she did not say a single word the whole time you were out."

"The whole time?" That's a long time to remain silent. I know it varied, the time it took me to wake up out of the anesthesia, but it was never less than seventy-five to ninety minutes from beginning to end.

"The whole time," my mother repeated. "In fact—and she told me I could tell you this—she cried the entire time. She cried, silently. Tears just rolled out of her eyes and didn't stop until you took that first breath on your own."

"I . . . I don't know what to say."

"I knew what she was feeling, and I told her that we were witnessing something sacred, something very spiritual."

"That if I attended any church, this would be it?"

My mom didn't laugh but gave me a gentle look. "No, it's so much more than that. Those people in that room have your life in their hands, and they don't have a machine telling them how much propofol to give you, or how far to take you down, or how long to keep you there. They are all working together as a team and trusting each other with the trust you have put in them."

We had talked about this before, this aspect of the treatment being so "human" in its machinations, but it took on so much more significance knowing that my sister had been there watching it play out. She got to see what I, the patient, did not.

"And given what her own kids have been through . . ." This is when my mother's voice began to crack. ". . . given what those kids have battled and worked to overcome and the sleepless nights your sister has stayed up worrying about whether or not they would pull through, I know this had deep meaning for her: that she is a mother and was there watching me with my own child, hoping you would pull through. You give her so much hope about her own kids."

My God, the crying. So much crying. I couldn't help but sit there and weep thinking about the struggle she had been through, the phone calls and text messages from her kids that probably resembled the phone calls and text messages from me to my mother. The same phone calls and text messages I am certain to receive from my own children.

"What you are going through is so sacred, Heather," my mom repeated. "To be in that room with you, to witness your bravery . . ."

"Is that what you really feel?" I asked through my tears. I did not feel brave. I felt like this was something I had to attempt, mostly for the sake of my girls. "I didn't have a choice, Mom. I had to do this. What else was I going to do?"

"Heather," she said and then she leaned forward, her elbows on her knees. "This is experimental. Read a description of what you're going through from the perspective of someone like your father." She had a point. "Your brother was mostly silent the whole time, too, although he did talk to Dr. Tadler a bit. You know what Dr. Tadler told Ranger?"

"Did he talk about the abyss?"

"He did, yes. But at one point he pointed to the monitor and said, 'See this point? About 40? When we take a patient's brain to here we can cut 'em.'"

"'We can cut 'em'?" I was confused.

"Surgery. When anesthesiologists get a patient's brain activity to that point, they can start cutting the body open. They're down far enough not to feel anything. And then he pointed to the bottom of the monitor and said, 'We are taking her all the way down.' When he put it like that, all of us gasped. We all knew, of course, but your brother put his hand over his mouth and shook his head in disbelief: the difference in what they do in surgery, and then what they are doing to you."

I pulled one of my giant throw pillows into my lap and hugged it like a teddy bear. What I was willing to do so that I could stop wanting to be dead. Period. I didn't want to feel that way, so desperately. *I did not want to feel that way,* and so I was willing to try or do anything. How is that brave? Is desperation brave?

"I was so desperate, Mom. You know how desperate I was."

"Yes, but you held on. You *held on*. You didn't give up. You didn't give in to this. You are a fighter and you came through."

"I did come through," I said as confirmation, for her and for myself. I had lived in an abyss for over eighteen months, and the abyss had brought me out of it. It had worked.

Later that night I put Marlo to bed. I have sung her the same four songs every night of her life after she reads and we turn off the lights—"Twinkle, Twinkle, Little Star," "Itsy Bitsy Spider," a verse from "The Little Drummer Boy," and a verse from "You Are My Sunshine"—and will continue to do so until she doesn't want me to sing to her anymore. When she is with her father, he does not sing to her because he thinks she's too old for that. Even if she is twenty-five years old and still finds comfort at night with my voice in her ear singing, "You make me happy, when skies are gray," you better believe I am going to whisper-sing that line into the velvety outline of her ear until she falls safely asleep. Because I am her mother.

I turned off her light and headed upstairs from her basement bedroom to watch an episode of *Felicity* with Leta. This nightly ritual we share has brought me closer to my daughter than anything else in our lives. We watch an episode of a show together every night— we started with *My So-Called Life* and graduated to *Felicity*. It has sparked conversations about topics ranging from love, abortion, marriage, divorce, romance, and what it's like to cram for finals in college. (Hint: It will destroy your ability to remember anything, especially faces and names.)

As I was walking up the stairs I got a text message. I turned on my phone to see who it was from. The rectangular white screen read "Ranger Hamilton." I opened it and looked down to read this:

"Today was a 'sacred' experience for me. Seeing you lying there, completely in the 0 abyss, I have never been more proud to be your brother. You have so much courage and so much fight in you. Your experience has now taken you to places I can't imagine. Please know that I say this next bit in total honesty—there were long-passed loved ones in the room watching over you. I felt them there and recognized them, as sure as I know I was there."

I had to lean against the countertop to steady myself. I knew exactly who he was talking about, the one person who immediately came to mind when Dr. Bushnell initially told me about the treatment. Her name was Minnie Ann McGuire, and she was my great-grandmother, the mother of my mother's mother. She bore nine children, two of whom died, and she spent the majority of her life in what was then referred to as a mental institution in Hopkinsville, Kentucky. My mother and her siblings have often posited that she suffered from ongoing postpartum depression that wasn't ever able to heal because she continued to get pregnant, and the deaths of two children only compounded her sorrow.

A journal entry written by Granny Boone while Minnie was still alive reads:

"Some day I'm sure my mother's mind will be healed and she will know the true gospel and she will be awarded according to her wonderful works in this life. The love I have for her can never be put into words on paper. When she reads this with a clear understanding may she find joy as I have found in writing it."

Tragically, Minnie spent her final days in that mental facility and died there in 1968. The nurses told my grandmother that they loved Minnie and that she was "the sweetest patient and the easiest to manage in the ward." Granny Boone once told one of my cousins, "Back then there were no counselors and therapists like there are today. They would just take them to Hopkinsville to the mental institution. Sometimes my mother would just sit for hours and stare. It seemed as though she was thinking. Sometimes she seemed emotionless. Other times she could be violent. At times she would lose her memory."

I had thought in the brief moments after learning about this treatment, *Will I be the one who ends up dying in a hospital?* Despite the immediate hope that the promise of the treatment had given me, I remember being struck by the idea that I was the craziest of all who had descended from Minnie Ann McGuire. Of course I was. Of course it'd be me. Heather, the Fuckup.

Her legacy is why I have fought so hard to get better each time my depression has reared its unforgiving head. Because back then there were no counselors and therapists like there are today. She didn't have access to the care and the help that I have access to, and she died long before she could ever get it. What was my eighteen months of hopelessness compared to the decades she spent locked inside an institution? All of this overcame me in that moment, especially the idea that here I was given another chance at life, *and it had worked.* If this long-passed loved one was in that room watching over me, I would want her to know that I think of her every time I reach for my bag of pills at night and how lucky I am to have them. Her legacy is the fight I have inside of me. Her legacy is a mother holding on for the sake of her two young girls.

SEVENTEEN

INTO THE INNER SANCTUM

I DON'T REMEMBER MUCH between the sixth and seventh treatments, only that my mother wanted to invite my father and stepmother to witness one before the study was over. Would I mind if they were in the room? I didn't see why not, only that everyone at the clinic would think, *Did she really bring an entire Southern state up here?* And I need to say this without it being read as unkind: my stepmother can sometimes make unintentionally hysterical commentary during, well, *always*. One of my first memories of her was in their living room in Arlington, Tennessee, where I was watching an early-morning news show. She passed through the living room, saw Bryant Gumbel interviewing some movie star, and said, "You know he looks just like a bar of milk chocolate. I kind of want to eat him." Not in jest, not with any sarcasm. It was just an observation she needed to make, out loud. I love this about her.

I was still managing to work half-time for the nonprofit that had been the source of so much of my anxiety. The day after the sixth treatment I saw my boss's name on my phone and I felt a giant pang of anxiety grip the upper half of my body. The treatment had cured me of wanting to be dead, but the Pavlovian jolts of anxiety would continue to be a side effect of my depression that I'd need to learn how to manage.

When I felt that raw emotion, I immediately called my therapist to make an appointment. I needed more encouragement from an outside party to help me leave the job. Managing my anxiety would mean I'd have to learn to say no and engage in conflict and pretty much reverse certain lifelong behaviors. If I quit that job, I'd be removing the biggest stressor in my life. Intellectually, I knew this. But I had tried once before and my boss talked me out of it. If you'll recall, I will apologize to you if you pee in my cereal because I will feel so bad that something in your life made you angry enough to do so, you poor thing. I couldn't get an appointment to see her for a few weeks, which was fine. I needed to die four more times anyway. Never a dull minute around here.

By the time I got in for my seventh treatment, I had fasted for over eighteen hours. If I'd known we were going to have to wait an extra hour after our arrival time, I would have taken a few swigs of water a little later than I had that morning. Luckily, Molly was the phlebotomist working that particular Wednesday. Unfortunately, the anesthesiologist listed on the whiteboard was the one who had let my eyes stay open during the entire fourth procedure, and this turned my mother up to eleven. I was warning Molly that I might be super-dehydrated, given that it had been so long since I'd last had any water, while my mother worked her way through the entire staff of the clinic to make sure that everyone there knew that my eyes needed to be taped shut, even people who did not need to know.

Molly and I were laughing about the bats in my vagina when Dr. Bushnell poked his head around the corner of the room.

"I thought I heard your laugh!" he said, his face a beam of sunshine.

"Hey!" I said. Since we hadn't yet gotten to the actual insertion of the needle, I jumped up to give him a hug, and he embraced me back.

As I sat back down, he took a seat next to the door, put his hand on his chin in a thoughtful pose, and said, "I heard you texted Dr. Mickey on Saturday. Hope you don't mind that he shared that with me."

"I don't mind at all!" I blurted. "I mean, I wanted to text the entire world, but I thought I'd start with him."

"He was happy that you reached out to him."

"Oh? Good. I didn't want to bother him on the weekend, but what I was feeling was just so significant that I thought he should know."

"It's good that you did. You know, there are no rules to this." Then he laughed. "We're making this whole thing up as we go along."

"Is that right," I said more than asked. Dr. Bushnell and I share the same sense of humor, so I had to bring him into this whole having-to-talk-about-my-sex-life nonsense. "Just so you know, I have to reveal each time during these needle intake interviews that I do not remember the last time I took my Macrobid prescription, meaning I don't remember the last time I had sex. Now everyone here knows that I am not getting laid. This isn't embarrassing or uncomfortable at all."

He chuckled and I prepared for him to respond in kind. "With the way you're glowing, Heather, I wouldn't be surprised if you showed up next time with a phone full of unsolicited pictures of men *in repose*, shall we say."

Dr. Bushnell looked over at Molly. "You see why we get along so well, yes?"

She nodded and smiled. I didn't tell either of them that I'd actually kissed someone for the first in ages, because they wouldn't understand the significance. I'd enjoyed being around someone, and although it technically hadn't been a date, I didn't want to flee. He hadn't made me feel like I wanted to die. And here several days later the feeling of that kiss lingered, if only because it had left me feeling hopeful.

"I'll let you get back to what you're doing," Dr. Bushnell said as he stood up. "I just couldn't resist the chance to say hello when I heard you. It's really good to see you like this." Then he walked over and squeezed my left shoulder before he left the room.

About an hour and a half later—after the gurney and the warm blanket and the Velcro wire and the giant vial of propofol and my mother's echoing refrain of "You are going to tape her eyes shut, yes?"—I woke up, blinked until I could focus, and exclaimed, "My mother married Satan, and when he's here next time you'll see *exactly* why she divorced him."

And then after my mother made sure I was feeling okay, I got my name right, and confidently told the nurse that the year was 1979. We did the usual awkward dance that had at this point become a ritual, as much a part of the treatment as the anesthesia itself. The numbers unfolded in my brain and I realized, *Oh, wait, it's 2017.*

As I came out of my drunken state, I turned to my stepfather, who was sitting to my left.

"Rob, I can't believe I just said that about my father. Along with taping my eyes shut, please have them tape my mouth shut when Dad is here. Oh my God."

"Are you kidding? I'm going to be standing right here next to you, provoking you with a cattle prod."

Later, in the early evening, my parents left. Marlo worked through her homework with Lyndsey, and Leta practiced piano. I sat down and entered the passcode on my desktop computer. I pulled up the email account for my nonprofit job and hit the red compose button. I didn't enter anything into the "To" or "Subject" lines and skipped directly to the body.

> Hey there, I want to talk about this in person, of course, but I need to give you a heads up that I have been going through something pretty heavy and important. And it has changed the trajectory of things for me. I can continue consulting for the remainder of this month and through the end of April, but after that I need to commit to some other projects for the sake of my mental health and my family. Although you convinced me to return the last time I announced my need to depart this work I really do need to head in a different direction. You know I have loved this work and truly believe in the mission of this organization. I have loved the professionalism and camaraderie I have shared with my coworkers, and the staff you've amassed is well-equipped to effect the change that has to happen with regards to the welfare of animals. Thank you for letting me be a part of it. I'd love to schedule a time to sit down and talk, so let me know what works best for you.

I wanted to get some words down now that I only had three treatments left. The looming end of the study made me feel an urgency. It wasn't a panicked or anxious urgency at all. It made me feel like I had the energy to start making the changes I needed to make. To take full advantage of the momentum of the light that I now felt on every part of my skin. I closed my eyes and immediately imagined the week ahead of me. There's that old cliché: "Today is the first day of the rest of your life." Whenever someone points that out earnestly, I feel like mauling them with a rake. We all know today is the first day of the rest of our lives, but that doesn't make whatever problem we were just agonizing about go away.

But what I felt right then, sitting at my desk and drafting an email to my boss giving notice—an email that would mean the end of a steady paycheck and months and years ahead of hustling to pay the bills—I felt like this was my second chance at life. It was such a glorious gift. The idea of losing that paycheck had fueled my anxiety for months, and now that thought no longer scared me. It no longer controlled me. It wasn't even a consideration.

I would not squander this gift.

I let the draft sit overnight so that I could read it the following morning with fresh eyes. It was a Thursday. I dropped off both girls at school, making the hour-long round trip first to the middle school and then to the elementary school while listening to music, marvelous, marvelous music. Then I sat down at my desk and read through the draft. Without changing a word, I entered my boss's email address in the "To" field and "March and April" in the "Subject" field.

When I hit SEND I felt a rush. I hadn't needed Mel's backup. I had entered into conflict willingly.

This was the beginning of the rest of my life.

———

The following morning my father and stepmother showed up at my house about twenty minutes before we needed to head to the clinic for my eighth treatment. They hadn't seen the house since they'd helped me move less than a month previously, and they wanted to have a look around. My mother and stepfather were already there, of course. All of my parents get along well, but we always experience an unacknowledged nervousness when all five of us are in the same room together. It stems from a fundamentally different way of looking at life. Even though all four are Mormon and staunchly conservative, my father and stepmother are more concerned about etiquette and formalities. That's not a wrong way to approach life, it's just different from my mother and stepfather. I don't have to worry that my very character is being judged if Marlo farts in front of my stepfather, even if she cups her hands around her butt and pretends to catch it. I didn't teach her this, although I wish I could take credit. If she were to do that around my father? I'd quickly rush her out of the room. When we have a holiday meal with my mother, we use paper plates. When we're at my father's house, we use ironed cloth napkins.

We made some small talk after they walked around and looked at each of the rooms—Marlo's and my own in the basement, Leta's room and my office on the ground floor just off the living room. This was by far the smallest house we had ever lived in. We once bought a 12,000-square foot house that I like to call the Beginning of the End of My Marriage, and I'm going to let you in on a secret: a big house does not bring happiness. You know what it might bring? Divorce! The smallness of this house was so surprisingly comforting that in the short time we'd been living in it Leta had declared that she'd never felt more at home. I felt exactly the same.

When it was time to leave, my father and stepmother got into their own car to follow us. I climbed into the back of the van like I always did and buckled into the seat, pilot-like, behind my mother. I forced myself to take in every smell and sight and movement of the van as we wound our way up to the clinic. I memorized the angle of the sun through the tint in the windows, the sounds of the construction sites we always passed. I knew that in a few years I would remember the apartment buildings going up and wonder about the people living inside of them. They wouldn't know that I'd driven by ten times, seeing the jackhammers and steel beams, on my way to get a second chance at life. Strange thoughts come to mind when you're in the midst of a life-changing experience. When you know you're inside of one, you don't want to take any moment of it for granted.

I will always remember the sway of the vehicle as it turned onto the curving Colorow Way toward the small parking lot filled with the vehicles of patients receiving ECT there. I will always remember the sound of the sliding door as I pulled it open to step out into the sun and feel it on my face, the buzz of a nearby generator greeting us. These details were so distinct to me, the same way your voice echoes when you reach the summit of a hike and yell an exclamation of victory.

Every time we walked toward the doors of the clinic, I would see our reflections in the full-length glass. That day I laughed, noting that I had gotten progressively cleaner and more fashionable with each passing treatment. I had showered and put on my favorite pair of jeans, a pair with a small hole on the right knee and a giant, gaping hole on the left. My father probably wondered why I was dressed so sloppily for something I had told him was so important to me, but he would never understand the significance of these jeans. How I had avoided wearing them for over eighteen months because they just didn't fit anymore, and what that feeling did to a woman who had been terrorized by the thought of food and eating throughout high school and college. I watched my left knee poke through the ragged hole with every step I took toward that door. They were the perfect item to wear to this important something.

All four of my parents took seats in the waiting room as I checked in and made small talk with Greg. Lauren once again said something nice about what I was wearing. Greg told me they were running slightly behind, not too far, but we'd need to wait at least twenty minutes. I glanced around the room, which was relatively full for that time of day. When I saw the faces of the other patients and those who had accompanied them, I thought, *Good. I'm glad we have to wait. My dad will have to sit here and be confronted with the reality of mental health and the toll it takes on people's lives.*

I'm sure that, for the first five treatments, if a stranger in that waiting room had looked at my face and into my hollow eyes, I would have looked like a corpse. You can't cover up a sincere desire to be dead with foundation or mascara or even a hoodie. And if someone who didn't really believe in the idea of depression had been sitting in that room, they'd have seen the looks on the faces of my mother and stepfather as well. It would have told a story of desperation and anguish, eighteen months of agony etched into three faces. I'd seen similar expressions on patients' faces while I waited. There were some in the room just then. Right there next to my father and stepmother, who were avoiding eye contact with anyone.

I took the seat next to my mother and leaned over to whisper, "We have to wait twenty minutes before I go get the needle in my arm. I'm kind of hoping for more if an unexpected patient shows up for the day." She chuckled under her breath, knowing exactly what I was getting at.

The television in the room was tuned to HGTV as it always was. All five of us watched a show about granite countertops.

None of us really said a word to each other. Usually we'd be discussing something that was going on in the family. But since so much of what was going on in the family was depression and we were sitting *right there* in the waiting room, with depression, despair, and hopelessness on the faces of multiple people around us, we all politely stared at the television. Finally they called for me to get the needle put into my arm. I returned about twenty minutes later. I nodded at my mother to indicate that they'd had to try more than twice to get the needle into a vein, and then I showed the bruises to my father.

"Whoa, Feather!" he bellowed as he leaned back to take it all in. He tilted his head so that he was seeing through the right part of his glasses and grabbed the arm where the needle was taped down to my forearm. "That has got to hurt. Who have you been fighting?" he laughed.

"These needles are not like normal needles," I explained. "They're bigger, more unwieldy. All the phlebotomists are getting used to them and I am the dummy they are using as practice."

"Can't they practice on a real dummy?" asked my stepmother.

"Well, I suppose they could if a real dummy had veins pumping blood," I said. "It's painful, but this really is the most uncomfortable part of the whole thing. So I can't really complain, not in the context of all that's happened."

Just then a nurse poked her head around the door and asked if we were ready. Most of the waiting room had cleared out by that point. Usually it was empty, and I wondered that day what those who were left were waiting for: Results? Paperwork? Relief?

I accompanied half of the state of Tennessee into the room where my gurney awaited me. Following all protocol, I confirmed my name and date of birth and gladly accepted the warm blanket a nurse handed to me before sitting down on the thin mattress. I looked over to see that my father and stepmother were sitting against the wall directly opposite me, and my mother and stepfather had taken places against the wall adjacent, to my left. As I reclined and swung my feet up on the mattress, I glanced at my father, who had at that point crossed his arms over his chest. My stepmother sat forward at the edge of her seat. At one point my stepmother started asking my mother questions, but because the team was assembling the vials and wires and paperwork, I didn't catch any of their conversation.

The procedure had become so rote at this point that I didn't try to resist the anesthesia. I knew it would take me away, that I had no power over it. All I remember is seeing the vial of propofol, that giant tube of milky-white fluid, and the tender look on my mother's face as I faded into nothingness. Yes, my heart was still beating, but my mother said that she took my stepmother over to the monitor to show her the abyss where my brain activity had been flattened. Friends would ask me if I ever saw anything—perhaps a light, or a tunnel, or any sort of dreamlike sensation—and my answer was always no. I saw nothing. There was black nothingness down there. I never felt them shove a giant breathing tube down my throat, heaving my body up and off the gurney in order to get it in at the right angle fast enough, which showed the depths of that nothingness.

I blinked, and in my blurry vision I could make out the glasses on my father's face as he sat next to me in the recovery room. Years of practiced repression enabled me to remain silent. I didn't say a word in my drunken state, and instead tried desperately to focus my eyes. My mother stood next to a nurse near the small refrigerator on the far wall, and my stepmother sat next to my father. She was clutching the neck of her sweater and looked confused. My father was expressionless, which didn't mean much: it is the resting state of his face. My stepfather sat next to Chris, and when I looked in their direction, my stepfather smiled at me. It was genuine and familiar and so comforting.

"Hey, glad you're awake," Chris said as he leaned a little toward my reclining body. I nodded. "Can you tell me your name?"

"I'm Heather B. Armstrong," I said distinctly. I was trying so hard to perform well for my father.

"Great," said Chris. "Now, can you tell me what year it is?"

I looked down at the blanket and concentrated on the shape of it as it draped over my feet. "It's 1979," I said, thinking my father would be impressed that I was getting all the answers right.

"Do you want to think about that a little more?" he asked.

Oh God. Had I gotten it wrong? The more I thought about it, the more certain I felt about it.

"But it's 1979," I said.

My stepfather smiled again, this time putting his head down. And then it all came back to me. All the times I had come out of anesthesia and spoken the wrong answer. Slowly the numbers began to crawl toward me. It wasn't 1993, no. I graduated high school that year. How about 1997? Graduated college that year. Then 2004 . . . 2007 . . . 2009 . . . 2012!

"Is it 2012?" I asked.

"Almost there," Chris said.

I closed my eyes and looked at the whole of my life in an instant. Two thousand and seventeen! God, why was this so hard?

"Two thousand and seventeen. Sorry, I don't know why this number gets away from me," I said to Chris. I hated that he had to work to get the right answer out of me.

A nurse I didn't recognize walked over and handed me a cup of apple juice that I slammed back in one gulp. She asked if I'd like another and I nodded. I wanted so desperately for my father to say something, anything, right then. But he was silent and motionless. Suddenly all I wanted in the world was to crawl into the back seat of that van. He had just witnessed what my mother had been witnessing over and over again. He knew that I wanted him to be there because of her and what this was doing to her. He had just watched my body go lifeless, his baby girl almost dead on a table. His silence said something so different than the silence of my sister.

Within a few minutes I felt steady enough to stand up. I swung my feet over the right side of the gurney so that my stepfather could help me. He made sure that I had my balance before we walked out into the hallway. The five of us, my Southern crew, walked in silence down the corridor toward the entrance. My father still said nothing. When we found ourselves outside in the sunlight on the black pavement of the parking lot, he quickly gave me a hug and told my stepfather to drive safely. That was it. My stepfather slid open the giant side door to the van so that I could climb inside, and he held my arm so that I didn't trip while doing so. This man. This man who so obviously loved me. This man who had given so much of his time and his life to this treatment, *for me*. He was giving himself to me. I had spent most of my adulthood supporting the men in my life, and here he was supporting me. And he was asking nothing in return.

As he slid the door shut behind me, I suddenly remembered my sixteenth birthday. My parents bought me a 1979 Datsun 510. It was gray, two-door, and had a stick shift. When they surprised me with it, I felt two very different emotions: (1) *Oh my God, they got me a car!* and (2) *Good lord, it looks like someone stepped on a cockroach and used a poop bag to scrape it off of their shoe.* My father drove me to a giant parking lot a few miles up the street to teach me how to drive the thing, because I had no idea what a clutch was.

My father apparently thought that the ability to drive a stick shift is something everyone is born with. We all come out of the womb able to breathe and suckle and shift into third gear. He was aggressive and urgent as he tried to explain how to start the car and shift gears, but I could not stop stalling the car as I tried to move it one inch forward. I couldn't get the damn thing moving, couldn't wrap my head around the tactics that made this machine operate. None of it made sense. The more I stalled the car, the more exasperated he became, and the more I stalled the car.

When he drove me home, I went straight to my room and cried into the pillows on my bed. About an hour later my stepfather knocked on my door and asked if he could try to teach me. We'd just take a spin around the neighborhood a few times, he said. He was so gentle about the offer that my desire to be able to drive the car overcame my blinding character flaw of avoiding anything for which I cannot be the valedictorian.

He drove me to the bottom of our street so that I wouldn't be attempting to shift gears on an incline. When I buckled in and took hold of the steering wheel, he said, "Just ease up on the clutch as you press down on the gas, as slowly as you need to. You'll feel it."

"But . . ." I was confused. "My dad said that if you don't pop your foot off the clutch that it will wear down really fast. And the last thing he wants to do is have to replace a clutch."

My stepfather laughed. "Yes, over the span of many, many years a clutch might wear out. Easing up on it as you start to drive is perfectly fine."

I turned the car on, pushed my left foot on the clutch as far down as it would go, then put my foot on the gas. I was holding my breath, and as I eased up on the clutch I could feel the car starting to move, and instinctively I knew when it was safe to ease all the way off of the clutch. The math clicked like the snap of two fingers. Within several hundred yards I was in second gear, within another hundred in third. We drove around the neighborhood for about fifteen minutes, and I didn't stall the car once. It just made sense. *Ease up on the clutch.* That was the secret.

My siblings and I have joked about this many times with each other. Both of them had to learn how to drive a stick under the tutelage of our father. They'd had, let's say, similar experiences to my own, although my brother's was true to form with his relationship with my father: the worst. Even my mother had to learn from my father, and she'd been so intimidated by his temper that she didn't learn to drive or get her license until she was well into her twenties. She later told me that as I left the house with him to drive to that giant parking lot, she wanted to reach out and save me. But *this was his thing*. He was our father and he was going to teach his children how to drive.

As my stepfather pulled out of the parking lot at the clinic, I couldn't help but think what a metaphor that experience was for what we'd been through over the previous three weeks. He was patient enough to let me ease up on the clutch. I know that if I had stalled the car all those years ago, he wouldn't have been irritated or angry or judgmental about my having been born helpless. Just like he'd been patient as he sat for hours with me at that clinic. In the waiting room, at the foot of my gurney as I lay there dying, he sat beside me as I came back to life. This man had given his love and patience to me in a way I had never experienced before, not even in a romantic relationship. Here this man was supporting me, and instead of fighting it and protecting the pride I'd built up through years of supporting myself, I was so happy to feel it and breathe it in.

"She talked the whole time," my mother suddenly exclaimed from the front seat.

"Who?" I asked.

"Your stepmother. She talked the entire time you were down."

"What did she talk about?"

"She kept asking questions. What was that thing for? Why was that noise going off? What does that line on the monitor mean? Why do they use a wire?"

"What about Dad? Did he say anything while I was down?" I asked, suspecting the answer.

My stepfather started shaking his head. "He sat there with his arms crossed the entire time. Didn't move. Didn't say a word."

"I wanted her to be quiet for just a minute to understand what she was watching," my mom continued, "to feel what we have felt each time watching you go into the depths. But it was as if they were there watching some ho-hum demonstration of something they didn't really understand."

"When they put the breathing tube in, did that startle her? Or Dad?"

"Yeah, that made her jump a bit. She asked why they were being so 'aggressive' with you, and I was, like, '*Because they are taking her brain to zero where she cannot breathe on her own!* And she is the valedictorian of getting to zero!' This was just the complete opposite of what it was like to have your sister and your brother there. Just completely different."

"Well, we kind of knew this might happen, right?" I asked, looking out the window. I admired the line the mountains cut into the sky.

"I just thought that if they could see it, they'd understand it at least a little bit more. And maybe they do. I'm sure I'll talk to them over the weekend. There was one thing, though . . ." she trailed off.

"What?" I asked.

"The way he sat there stroking your forehead before you woke up."

"Wait, what?" I hadn't remembered this gesture.

"Your father, he sat next to you after they wheeled you into the recovery room. He stroked your forehead with his thumb for the entire hour it took you to wake up. You don't remember this?" she asked.

I shook my head. I didn't remember a single second of it. And I could hardly believe it.

"He didn't say anything, and it was almost as if he were remembering your childhood. That was the look on his face. Maybe that's the only way he knew how to respond, to try to comfort you in some way." Maybe he, too, remembered once lifting me over his shoulders to reach up high into the trees. Maybe that gesture was his way of saying, "I don't understand any of this, but I'm here."

Later that night my brother would call my mother to tell her that they'd had my father and stepmother over for dinner. All night long my stepmother expressed concern about what she'd witnessed. What had Heather gotten herself into? And this made my mother sad that she had invited them into our sacred space. It felt instead like an invasion.

I hadn't been awake to witness the bulk of it. I only sensed the distance when I woke up. I felt like I needed to comfort my mother. We'd hoped it would open their eyes, and we invited them with the best of intentions. But now we knew for sure; we wouldn't talk to them about our own struggles, and especially not about the struggles of our children. We'd come too far in recognizing the signs and symptoms of depression in our family. None of us should have to deal with someone questioning whether or not our suffering was real.

When we arrived home after that treatment, the kids were inside watching a movie. They get out of school early on Fridays. Leta immediately paused the show, jumped up, and ran to hug me.

"Do you need us to be quiet so that you can take a nap?" she asked.

I didn't feel tired, oddly enough. I shook my head. As she ran back to the couch, I turned to my stepfather who had stepped inside behind me. They didn't need to stay and I didn't want to take up any more of their day, not another minute of their time. I told them I was good, that they could leave. Then I reached up and embraced my stepfather like I never had before. We'd hugged before, of course. My mother and he have been married for over thirty years; there have been many, many hugs. But something had changed, as recently as that treatment. I love my dad; I don't think I have to qualify that. He's never balked at helping my mother financially with us, his children. He's lived up to his duties to us as someone who chose to bring us into this world. I know he loves us. But now I also know the love of a father who loves me despite the endless differences between us, who dedicated himself to me, showed up and was present and understood and believed and held gently in his palm the silent, ticking moments as my lifeless body rested on that gurney—*When will she breathe on her own again? Will she breathe on her own again?*—to drive me there and back home, each time, over and over. It was unlike any love any man had ever shown me.

My stepfather had witnessed what my phone calls had done to my mother emotionally, the toll my treatments were taking on her physically. He didn't hold any of it against me, and he'd be back again on Monday to do it all over again. I lingered for a moment in the hug and then pulled back to look him directly in his eyes.

"I love you, Rob. Thank you. Thank you for all that you have given me. You are such an amazing father."

EIGHTEEN
WEEKLY SUNDAY PANIC ATTACK

I SPENT THE WEEKEND huddled with my children inside our small home. It rained for two days straight, an odd occurrence in a semi-arid state. Showers are usually brief and infrequent or they just turn into snowstorms. I was thrilled that this rain was not turning into snow, although being stuck in a confined space with a bored seven-year-old and a moody thirteen-year-old was the perfect way to test whether or not I still wanted to be dead. Add in a dog who sat at the door and barked if the wind blew—a bark so jarring that it sent a jolt up my spine—and suddenly I was yearning to be on a gurney staring at a vial of propofol.

During the previous eighteen months of my depression, Sundays had become the worst day of the week by far. My boss had instated a protocol for the whole team that required us to track the projects we were working on in a document. He wanted a detailed, line-by-line reckoning of the work we were doing, and he wanted it first thing

Monday morning. Updating that document made performing my duties even more loathsome. At the end of the day, as kids piled into the house and the raucous noise of the afternoon routine began, I'd realize that I hadn't updated that document. I'd jot down a few notes so that I could write everything up later.

I'd wake up on Sunday mornings and be seized first with the idea of that document and second with the idea that we were going to have to start the week all over again and address All of the Things Needing to Get Done.

This Sunday I woke up and was seized once again with the idea of that document, even though I had already given my notice. This feeling confirmed that I'd made the right decision. I had to eradicate this cancer from my life in order to start managing my anxiety. I then thought about the last two treatments, how I was going to have to starve myself two more times. Fortunately, this de facto intermittent fasting had decreased my appetite. Still, I can testify that it's never fun to go almost twenty hours without eating.

Leta woke up in a terrible teenage mood yet again, and by early afternoon Marlo's boredom had reached a fevered pitch. I was holding it together and breathing through the frenzied thoughts I was having, when I realized that I needed to write it down. Something about writing it down would calm me, and one ingredient in that day's panic was the pending relaunch of my website. I needed to start writing again. In a therapy session a couple of months prior, Mel had helped me realize that I had used my blog for well over a decade to work through my feelings. Writing had proven to be an effective therapy for processing confusion and frustration. Not having that outlet had contributed to this episode of depression. I needed to start writing again, and having an audience had always been a huge motivator.

After convincing Leta to play *Minecraft* with Marlo—"convincing" here meaning offering money—I sat down at the kitchen counter to text my mother:

> I know you won't get this until later, but writing this down will help me. Marlo's boredom and frustration are a huge trigger for me. She experiences massive swings in mood when she "doesn't have anything to do." Leta is also exhausted and grouchy. I think I just feel so alone in having to remain calm and maneuver around their feelings while indexing in my head the amount of work that lies in front of me this week. It's terrifying. This is the crux of my anxiety. Is this just my fate as a single working mom? I think it is and this makes me feel like I have so much work to do on how I cope. Just know that I am trying to explain why I'm so anxious about the upcoming week. I have to starve myself on Monday and Wednesday and I'm supposed to launch my website by Friday while working another full-time job. While navigating irritable, bored children. Hi, this is my weekly Sunday panic attack.

About ten minutes later she responded:

> Your responsibilities as a single mother are completely overwhelming. Rob and I are driving home from church and should be done with dinner by 6. I can talk any time after that. Also, we are coming to take the girls to Chick-fil-A on Tuesday night after I do your laundry. Do not argue with me. END OF DISCUSSION.

She signed it with her usual blue heart, blue because that is the school color for BYU.

I called her at about 6:30 with the sound of rain pounding against the awning on the front porch. I'd just finished adding two single-spaced pages of details on the work I'd been doing for the nonprofit. It was work I was jamming in before and after treatments, and I sent the document off to my boss. The sense of relief bordered on ecstasy. That was done. I'd only ever have to do four more of them. And then I'd be free to find something else to panic about.

My mother listened as I again listed the reasons why I was so anxious. As I spoke, I realized that all of what I was feeling was rooted in urgency, not sadness. I was overwhelmed, yes, but not hopeless. I'd unloaded the dishwasher earlier in the day without thinking that doing so would make my hands fall off, and even said to my mother, "I can't believe how utterly devastating it used to feel when I knew I'd have to unload the dishwasher again. It would destroy me. That sounds so stupid, but I *felt* it. The feeling consumed me. I can't tell you how happy I am to be free of that, to see a simple chore and not be immediately overcome by despair."

She pointed out that I was expressing happiness during my weekly Sunday panic attack, and that maybe this was a good sign. And it was! This renewed feeling of wanting to be alive made me see that I needed to manage my responsibilities to my kids and to my job more effectively. Now that I was out of that hole, I could go about the work of doing so. And there in the middle of my weekly Sunday panic attack, I heard Marlo giggle over something she had built in *Minecraft* with the best older sister she could have asked for. I felt oddly optimistic, and it was thrilling to experience that emotion.

NINETEEN
THE FINAL HOURS OF SUMMER CAMP

THE NINTH TREATMENT WASN'T noteworthy in any way other than the fact that it was still pouring outside. That month of March would end up being the wettest March on record for the state of Utah. When I heard that, I dramatically imagined it as a metaphor for what we'd all lived through. A cleansing. I'd worked all morning on the redesign of a website encouraging institutions that serve food to source from farms with high standards of animal welfare. I should note here that I'd added a little bit of meat back into my diet a few weeks before I started treatment and immediately felt a difference in satiation and bloating. I decided that never again would I run another marathon while subsisting on mung beans and kale. I also decided that I'd never run another marathon, period.

Just like we had eight times before, the three of us climbed into the giant minivan, wound our way up to the clinic, and took our places in the waiting room. I nodded happily at Greg as he handed me the clipboard. When I sat down with it, I just wanted to draw a giant X on both sides of the paper and write, "Despite some ongoing anxiety around work and running my household *I feel fantastic!*" After a phlebotomist stabbed me several times in the arm, I headed toward my gurney, my mother and stepfather walking behind me. And then the warm blanket, Velcro wire, lidocaine, propofol, and all of the formalities. The bliss of total nothingness. The abyss. When I woke up, I looked around through the blurriness of my sight and finally focused on Chris. Before he could say anything, I blurted, "I've been taking showers." As if he would understand the significance of this instead of thinking, *Well, that is the worst come-on I've ever heard.*

But it was true. I'd been regularly taking showers and applying mascara. A few times a week I'd even apply a foundation, some eye shadow. I was wearing jeans and shirts one doesn't wear to a spin class. My kids were coming home from school, seeing my clean hair and my outfit, and wondering what was going on. I sat down to watch *Felicity* that night with Leta, and before she started the show and leaned into my lap, I asked her if we could talk.

"Yeah," she said, surprised. Usually we have our in-depth conversations *after* the show sparks inevitable conversations about all the complexities of life. "Is everything okay?"

"That's kind of what I wanted to talk to you about," I answered. "Everything is great. Really good, in fact."

"I didn't want to say anything," she said. "Did . . . did what you're doing . . . did it work?"

"Yes. Yes, it did," I said. "I feel so much better. I can breathe so much more easily now."

"Like . . ." It felt like she was trying to be as gentle as possible. "Like, last week. Last week especially. It was like . . . I don't know . . . things were less intense, you know?"

"I do. I know."

"Like, Grandmommy wants me and Marlo to be quiet when you're sleeping, but you didn't sleep as much. And you seem, like . . . like, a lot more relaxed."

"Do I?" I wanted to laugh at this particular observation, but I didn't. I know that everyone around me could feel my anxious state, and no one could feel it more intensely than she did. That was nothing to laugh about.

"Yeah, like you've been completely different. Smiling and laughing and . . . like, things seem different."

"You know I wanted to get better. I've wanted to get better for a long time." She nodded and then suddenly shot out her arms and embraced me, resting her head on my right shoulder. I stroked her hair and took in her scent. "I'm so sorry it's taken so long. I'm really sorry. I know it's been hard. I'm so, so sorry."

"It's okay," she said into my shirt. "I know you have so much to do. Like, you're doing all of this alone."

"I do a lot of it alone," I agreed. "But Grandmommy and Grandpa Rob have helped so much. I couldn't have done this without them. And you help out so much. You know that, right?"

"I do? How? You have to drive me to school and dance and piano, and sometimes I get into those moods. I'm sorry—"

"No, you are not to blame here. You are not the culprit."

"But—"

"No, Leta. It's my brain. I needed to jump-start my brain somehow." I tried to figure out a way to describe it to her. "It's like my brain got caught in the middle of the ocean with no raft and it could only tread water before it got too tired and too weak to keep moving its arms and legs. And then at some point it couldn't move them at all. We had to send in a rescue boat as it started to sink. And I guess you could say that it almost drowned before we got there. And I'm so happy we got there. You are included in that 'we,' because you work so hard and are the best sister to Marlo. You are so good to her, and that helps me so much."

"It does?" she asked.

"You have no idea," I answered. "You play with her and read with her, and you help me remind her of the things she's supposed to be doing as an active citizen of this world. Has she forgotten her lunch once this year?"

"Has she?"

"Not once! You help me remind her as we're walking out the door in the morning, and even that one little thing has relieved my burden."

"I'm so glad it worked, Mom. I was worried."

"I know you were, and I am so sorry. But you don't have to worry anymore. I'm so glad it worked, too."

———

Two days later, on the afternoon of March 29, 2017, my parents showed up to take me to my last treatment. The solemnity of those hours was lost on none of us. To break the heaviness of the silence after they walked in my door, I clapped my hands together and said, "I certainly could use one more trip to the land of the dead!"

"You're awful," my mother said.

I have talked to them about this since, so I can say with confidence that the three of us were experiencing a shared melancholy. We were like friends who've attended a summer camp together and have to say goodbye. Not that I was saying goodbye to them, but we had endured something together so profoundly binding that the idea of it ending almost physically hurt. This would be our last drive up the winding streets; the last time we'd sit together in that waiting room seeing the faces of others whose features had been disfigured by hopelessness; the last time I would have to feel the jolt of a needle shoot up my arm and into the bottom of my jaw. It would be the last time I'd look over to see the relief on my stepfather's face when he realized my mother had found an audience in me for her constant chatter.

And then as I lay on the gurney, the wire affixed to my forehead, the warm blanket tucked over my body and between my arms, I looked at each and every face around the room. The research assistant, my stepfather, my mother, two nurses, a woman anesthesiologist named Dr. Whittingham, and Dr. Mickey. Before Dr. Whittingham began to show me the vials of liquid, I had to say something.

"Dr. Mickey!" I shouted.

He'd been staring down at a notepad and looked over at me. When he saw the intense look on my face, he walked toward me. As he stood directly at my side, I gave him a huge smile.

"Thank you," I said. "Thank you for giving me my life back."

"I'm just happy that you feel better," he said with a smile, and then he began to blush. Taking compliments always seemed a little awkward for him. "That's what we're trying to do here."

I looked around the room again. "Thank you, all of you. My girls got their mother back. You gave me back to them. Thank you." When Dr. Bushnell told me a week later that everyone working on me was donating their time, I was stunned. I will not ever get over that. I will not ever be able to repay that generosity. I can only speak it out loud and write it in words and remember them each time I sing Marlo a song as she goes to sleep. Because of them I am still alive and able to sing to my child at night.

Dr. Whittingham asked if I was ready, and I nodded. Ready

for my last ride into the vast darkness, all-consuming and calm. An unmoving pool of blackness free from worries and thoughts and the agonizing struggle to keep up with the relentless pace of life up above. Blissful nothingness. The healing abyss.

I relished the last few moments as Dr. Whittingham held up the vial of propofol. I memorized the shape and color of the room. As she told me she was beginning the anesthesia, I looked over at my mother's face and nodded. She nodded back, both of us knowing what she was feeling and what I was feeling. And then . . . nothing.

The final dive to zero.

Then suddenly I was awake. I was alive and breathing on my own. No longer would my mother have to wonder if my chest would move with my first breath on that gurney. Ten treatments done, experiment completed. In my final drunken state I remained silent, somehow still gripped by the sacred aspect of having received this gift.

When the nurse asked me what year it was, I quietly answered, "It's 1979." And I had no idea why my mother started laughing.

TWENTY

MY CALLING

A COUPLE OF WEEKS later I was sitting across from Mel. The orange tassels of the blanket were draped across my legs. I was resuming our weekly sessions at 3:00 p.m. on Wednesdays now that the treatment was over. She had a smirk on her face and was waiting for me to say something. I just sat there smiling and rubbing my right temple because *where do I even begin?*

"Well?" she asked.

"It's like that Adele song except it's not a downer at all. It's like Adele broke up with an abusive and narcissistic asshole, and she's like, 'Hello from the other side—*bye!*'"

"You're cracking me up," Mel said.

"And she is not sorry, not one little bit. And the hell if she picked up the phone to dial his ass ever again."

I tried to sum it all up without gushing about all the tiny details that would mean nothing to anyone else. Things like Greg's sneakers and Lauren's hair color and how it felt to hold the clipboard in my hand as I asked myself just how much I wanted to be dead and the moment I looked at that questionnaire and realized a switch had been flipped. Looking up and seeing my stepfather in the front seat of the enormous van, sacrificing his day because he loved me so much. My mother running around the clinic to make sure everyone followed protocol: no fentanyl, no Zofran, warm blanket, tape her eyes shut, apple juice stat! Swapping labor stories with Molly and the feel of the giant needle entering my arm and confirming repeatedly that my sex life had not yet resumed. How Dr. Mickey was a man of few words even though he was the one who had pulled this treatment together and convinced all those wonderful people to volunteer their time. Arguing endlessly with Chris about whether or not it was 1979.

"I'm so good," I said, "that I'm seeing someone *here in Utah* and he doesn't make me want to be dead."

"Are you kidding me?" she asked. She'd endured hours of my online dating stories and tried to help me work through why I was attracting that kind of frustration into my life.

"Yeah, it's nothing too serious. He's a musician, sort of, and by day and sometimes through the night he works on film sets. We've seen each other a few times."

"What do you like about him?"

"Well, he has a job! My God, my bar is so low. We share a common Mormon and Southern heritage, which is always nice to have. He's a little wacky, and it's kind of cute. But this *thing* happened after my last treatment."

"What do you mean?"

"Well . . . my parents took my kids to dinner for the second night in a row so that I could get some work done. He texted me and asked if he could stop by and say hello. Since the kids were gone I told him to come over and, I don't remember why, but I had run downstairs to get something from my room when he started to play some chords on the piano. You can't escape the piano in that house. And I was about to walk back upstairs when he began playing the first few lines of a song by the Cure. And I froze. I totally froze. I couldn't believe it, I was in total shock. Because that song—it's called 'Trust'—is a song I used to play on repeat in high school when David Smith broke my heart. *David Smith*, oh my God. In eleventh grade David compared me to Dominique in *The Fountainhead* so I read it and fell in love with him. This is so embarassing."

Mel started to laugh a little.

"I *know* I am a totally dramatic hag, but hear me out."

"I'm sorry: Go on."

"Sure, I was a moody teen and just had my heart shattered into a million pieces, but you and I both know that I was so depressed in high school. I just didn't know it was depression."

"You've been depressed since your childhood," she confirmed, almost as if to remind me.

"Right. So, this song—I played it on repeat for months and months. I'd lie on the floor in my bedroom in total darkness and just cry. This song was the soundtrack to my depression."

"Did he know this? The guy you're seeing?"

"NO! That's just it. Of all the songs in the world to pluck out on a piano, of all days? *That day?* I haven't heard that song in at least a decade, if not longer. He was playing the soundtrack of my depression on the last day of a treatment that had healed the worst episode of depression in my life."

"That's pretty wild," she agreed.

"I'm not gonna get all woo-wooey about this, but shit is happening, Mel."

"Go on."

"I'm going to Paris."

She shook her head in confusion.

"I remember sitting on my porch after that fifth treatment when I texted Dr. Mickey to thank him. And I was suddenly overcome with the thought that more people need to know about this. This whole thing could save so many lives."

She nodded and was waiting for me to elaborate.

"And I know that you and I and my mom, we were all afraid that Jon would find out about this—about how bad my depression was—but this is too important. I want to write a book about it."

"Okay, first, this is what you were meant to do. That you have arrived at this conclusion on your own is huge. Two, who cares if Jon finds out? We do not care anymore."

"I did arrive at this conclusion on my own, yes. But one afternoon my mother could tell that I was waffling about quitting the nonprofit— Oh! by the way, I quit the nonprofit. I was going to wait to get a pep talk from you, but I died ten times instead. I am so happy to be alive that I quit my job! And I'm not experiencing any second thoughts. I asked myself, *What would my therapist tell me to do?* And I did *that*."

"HEATHER!" she shrieked.

"I know! But wait! We were waiting to leave for my seventh treatment and my mother could sense my hesitation. I mean, money is a trigger for me. I had to decide if that steady paycheck was worth the ongoing panic attacks, and as I was talking through that with her, she looked me squarely in the eyes and said, 'Look at me. Your calling is not with those cows.' And I started laughing because she sounded like she was really angry at cows. But then I realized she was on the verge of tears. She was, like, 'Your calling is with your sister whose children suffer from something she cannot possibly understand, and you are giving her a peek into their worlds. Your calling is with her children who now have a mom who has a reference point, who has words she can put to what they are feeling.'"

"So, you're going to Paris to write, aren't you?"

"Yeah. I am. The girls will spend half of their summer in New York with Jon, so why not take some time for myself and write?"

"Heather, this is the best idea you've ever had. Other than agreeing to that treatment, of course. Bravo. Standing ovation."

"Thank you. It was an easy decision to make. Things are just *easier*. I don't know how to explain it."

"You're more relaxed, that's why. And the change in your face is so dramatic that it says to me that shit is happening because you are putting out a completely different energy."

"That's just it! I am! I mean, I was on the phone with AT&T, telling the customer service representative where I was going. She was making friendly small talk and asked if I was going with anyone. And when I told her that, no, I was going to Paris to be alone and write, she asked me what I was going there to write about. And I was, like, *oh no. Womp-womp*. Here's where things are going to get awkward. So I told her, 'It's a book about depression.' And, Mel, I mean . . . she perked right up and asked me about my own depression before launching into a forty-five-minute description of the months she spent battling suicidal ideation, how her *daddy* stepped up and saved her from it. And by the end of the phone call we were both crying. Because my stepdad did the same thing for me. *An AT&T representative, for God's sake.*"

"That's what a dad is supposed to do," she reminded me.

"Yes. I know that now. There's so much I know now. These people keep coming out of the woodwork, people I do not know, to talk to me about how depression has affected their lives. Over and over again I keep finding myself in these conversations. Just . . . from out of nowhere. And not a single one of them has batted an eyelash when I tell them what I just went through."

"How could they? Look at you. I've never seen you so inside of your body before. So alive. You have color in your face. And your eyes, Heather: when you walked in, your eyes told me that you'd robbed a candy store and were not worried one bit that you'd be caught."

I laughed under my breath and sat there taking all of this in.

"You have to promise me a couple of things," she said, and I could tell she was serious. "This book . . . no one knows how afraid you were about losing your kids, do they?"

I shook my head.

"You're going to write about that in this book. Single parents need to hear that coming from you. Single parents who don't even suffer from depression fear this all too often. I talk to them every day of the week. Your calling is with them, too. Don't forget that."

"Okay," I agreed, and nodded.

"And your father—"

"Oh God, wait—"

"Hear me out. You and your mom and your sister and your brother all tiptoe around him like he's some sort of land mine just waiting for you to step right on top of it. You know I think you should jump on it like a trampoline, but he's the father out there you're trying to reach. How many other fathers out there refuse to accept the supposed shortcomings of their children? Not that depression is a shortcoming—"

"I know what you're saying."

"Those children out there need to hear it from you, too. You are living their experience. You've lived it your entire life."

I nodded. And then I began silently sobbing for all the children out there whose parents don't believe them. We so desperately do not want to feel alone.

We don't want to feel this way.

We would do anything not to feel this way. The lengths we will go to so that we no longer feel this way. I sat there crying for those of us who believe the only way out is through death, wishing we all had someone like my mother who chooses to listen and believe. I cried harder for those of us who don't, who do not ever make it up and out of the hole. I cried for those of us stuck in the loop of the lie, that the world would be so much better off without us.

Please believe us.

Help us find our way up and out and back to the truth that you would not be better off without us.

EPILOGUE

AS OF AUGUST 2018, I haven't experienced any sort of relapse or bout of depression in eighteen months. I haven't had a single thought resembling, "It would be nice to be dead right now." In fact, I still feel like I've been given a second chance at life. I'm still hopeful. I'm energetic, and dare I say this out loud? I'm *happy*.

Recently, I interviewed Dr. Mickey in his office a few blocks away from the ECT clinic at the University of Utah. This was the first time I had seen him since I ended treatment. The fact that my bout of suicidal depression had lasted eighteen months—and that eighteen months later I was able to sit across from Dr. Mickey feeling whole and good and *happy*—will not ever be lost on me.

His blond hair still looked boyish, and when he spoke I remembered how gentle he had always been during our conversations. I was asking him to explain some of the more technical aspects of the treatment.

"Can you tell me more about 'the abyss,' what exactly that means you're doing to someone's brain?"

"The BIS, yes," he answered.

"No, I mean, 'the abyss,' " I clarified. "My mother took a picture of the lines on the monitor during one of my treatments to show me the line indicating my brain activity. And when it was near zero you called it 'the abyss.' "

"Well, the monitor itself is called a BIS. B-I-S. It stands for bispectral index," he clarified. "It's an EEG-type of machine that gives feedback to an anesthesiologist. We used that machine to target the propofol treatments, since we were using a level that is far deeper than what anyone would receive for any kind of surgical procedure."

He continued to explain the state of burst suppression that he and the anesthesiologist tried to achieve with each treatment. I'm relieved that I recorded our conversation, because all I could concentrate on was the thought that my mother had misheard him while I was under anesthesia during my first treatment. She thought he had pointed to the line on that monitor lingering at the very bottom and called it "the abyss." That term made so much sense that I never questioned it. In fact, "the abyss" became so emblematic of the journey that I took with my mother through ten treatments that I had it engraved on a gold bracelet that I gave her on Mother's Day.

When I left Dr. Mickey's office, I immediately texted her: "You're going to want to sit down for this."

I also found out that morning that Dr. Mickey and his team had completed the first round of the propofol study. It included ten pa-tients, all of whom received ten treatments over the course of three weeks. Of those ten—the only ten people in the history of humanity to receive propofol in this way—he said that six experienced a positive response. That included me, the third patient. Of those six, five continued to experience positive effects after three months. I don't know how those other five people continue to feel, but eighteen months after completing this experimental study I still feel exactly as I did when I looked at that questionnaire after the fifth treatment. Had I really wanted to be dead?

When I asked Dr. Mickey how he felt about the results of the study he said he was encouraged. "As a scientist you have to be very self-critical, that's part of your job," he said. "You have to be very circumspect about other possible explanations for what we saw. The results were pretty impressive, though, when you've treated a lot of people with treatment-resistant depression. These are the kinds of results that we see with ECT. We see a high response rate, usually very quickly."

Those other explanations, he told me, included things like the natural history of the disease—many depressive episodes will end on their own because they are situational. There's also the placebo effect to consider, as well as all the attention a patient is suddenly receiving from medical staff and family members. There's even the fasting aspect to preparing for the treatment itself. He said, "When you get these treatments you have to fast three time a week. Fasting three times a week for three weeks, does that have antidepressant effects? We don't think so. We think that's unlikely, but we don't *really* know."

I'm not fasting three times a week anymore. I'm no longer spending that much time with my mother and stepfather, and I still have a list of All the Things Needing to Get Done that doesn't ever get done.

I know that my depressive episode wasn't going to end on its own, and I'm confident that without this treatment I would still want to remain forever in the abyss. My life is as chaotic and unmanageable as it has ever been, and I am handling it.

Dr. Bushnell now requires that I see him every three months for a checkup, and at this checkup he writes the refills for all my prescriptions. I take six different medications to manage my depression, including the original cocktail that treated my insomnia. I took all six during the treatment. Dr. Bushnell changed a couple of the antidepressants I was on because certain medications can lose their effect due to hormonal changes, physiological changes, age, and a myriad other reasons. When it was over he emphasized the importance of staying on my medication to help prevent any deterioration in my mental health. I don't have any problems following this order. Although that may sound like a lot of medication to take every day, I feel happy now—I'd gladly take double that amount, if necessary.

I have in the last eighteen months been invited to run several long-distance races for various worthwhile causes, and every time I have experienced no hesitation when declining the offer. Part of the ongoing "medication" for my mental health has been identifying triggers for my anxiety. I either avoid these triggers altogether or I develop habits to handle them. I have developed better ways of thinking about life. The treatment got my brain back to a place where I could start making these cognitive changes. This includes asking for help, *all the time*. I have no doubt that one major contributing factor to my happiness is the teenager I hired to help Marlo practice piano.

I used to think I was good at choosing my battles. What that depressive episode taught me was that I was terrible at it. In order to manage my anxiety, I have to let so much go. This isn't easy for a valedictorian. I have to practice letting go every single day, and it's hard. But I do it—for myself, and the people I love, and on behalf of everyone who is fighting for their lives.

AFTERWORD

Brian J. Mickey, MD, PhD

YOU'VE BEEN STRUCK BY a debilitating brain illness. A cardinal symptom of this particular disease is the inescapable urge to kill yourself, fueled by a loss of hope. Even in the face of these symptoms, you have somehow managed to diligently attempt multiple treatments that were recommended by your doctors, to no avail. You, along with tens of millions of other individuals around the world, have treatment-resistant depression.

One of my roles as a psychiatrist who specializes in this illness is to provide hope. And there is indeed reason for hope. We have in our toolkit more evidence-based medications and psychotherapies for depression than ever before. Recent decades have brought new brain stimulation therapies such as transcranial magnetic stimulation. Furthermore, refinements of the oldest and most effective brain stimulation intervention in psychiatry—electroconvulsive therapy—have reduced its side effects and established it as one of the safest medical procedures.

Yet, these various options still leave us wanting. For most of these potential interventions, success rates remain at or below 50 percent. In addition, side effects prevent many from trying or continuing these treatments. Adding insult to injury, poor access, inadequate reimbursement, stigma, and public misunderstanding are barriers that we encounter every day. These various challenges amplify each other, leading to lengthy depressive episodes that can go on literally for years.

This situation has inspired scientists like myself to search for new treatments that work in a different way. If these novel interventions are sufficiently different, they might be more effective or better tolerated than current treatments. This is the stage on which the propofol study plays out.

Clearly, Heather Armstrong is no ordinary study volunteer. She brings her individual story to life with her own unique and compelling voice. Heather does, however, have two things in common with the other participants of the propofol study. First, she was struck by this debilitating illness whose causes remain mysterious. Second, despite the illness—or perhaps because of it?—she bravely volunteered to undergo an unproven intervention in the hope of advancing medical science.

It is important to emphasize that Heather knew that proven treatment options were available to her—albeit with the limitations described above. She was also well aware that propofol had never been tested in humans for this purpose. Although our team had reasons to believe that propofol might have antidepressant effects, we were essentially working off a scientific hunch. And she was aware that, while we considered the procedure to be quite safe, there was still a small risk of serious injury or death.

Put in a similar situation, would you volunteer? Perhaps you would feel inspired by the potential to generate new knowledge that could someday help others. It is possible that you would trust the study team, the scientific institution, and the sponsor. Maybe you would be able to push through your symptoms, or push them away long enough, to sign that consent form and bravely step into the unknown, as Heather did.

The study Heather participated in could be the beginning of something new. But the true benefits of propofol for treatment-resistant depression remain unknown. Much work still needs to be done.

ACKNOWLEDGMENTS

I would like to thank my editor, Jeremie Ruby-Strauss, who resisted every urge to ask, "You did *what?*" when I called to tell him that I wanted to write this book. Without his faith in this story I know that I would still be knocking on doors trying to convince someone that a switch had flipped. He has been both my champion and my advisor, and he is to thank for the glaring lack of sentences written entirely in caps lock in these pages. I have sent him flowers on your behalf.

Many thanks to the team at UNI who took such good care of me, including Dr. Brian Mickey and Dr. Scott Tadler. I owe my psychiatrist, Dr. Lowry Bushnell one, if not both, of my kidneys. He put it this way: I won the lottery. I happened to be sitting in his office when Dr. Mickey was looking for another patient for this trial. How lucky I was to be number three out of tenin the world.

I am indebted to my talk therapist Mel for guiding me through the darkest months of my life and trusting that I had something inside of me that would hold on for my girls. Because of her I can now eat chips and salsa with a smile.

I also want to thank Simon Wheatcroft for guiding *me* to the finish line of the 2016 Boston Marathon and Karen Walrond for modeling what it means to be a woman who could look at item 11 on the How Much Do I Want to be Dead Assessment—the item asking me to determine my view of myself—and think, *I run this world*. A thank you to Roxanna Sarmiento whose compassionate glance toward me over a meal in Pattaya, Thailand, told me that what I had confided in her about my crippling appetite was heard and seen and trusted. Thanks also goes to Michael Lopp who in February 2016 asked me over a drink in Wellington, New Zealand, what I wanted most in life. I'd never considered it before he asked me, and the day after my fifth treatment when I was sitting on my porch watching my children ride their scooters back and forth I remembered that conversation. I had answered, "I want to be still. I want to watch my children be children."

My most sincere gratitude goes out to John Bray for hearing the sadness in my voice and always checking in on me, to Stacia Sidlow for stroking my hair the night I needed it most, to Ivy Earnest for stepping in as my sister wife and hosting sleepovers for my girls. Many thanks to Ivy and Josh for loving my kids as their own.

A special thank you is owed to Jordan Ferney who convinced me that Paris isn't just some ordinary European town. Without her encouragement I would have never booked my three-week stay in the city where this book came alive, in the city where *I* came alive. I could write a library of gratitude for Paris and what it gave to me, but the shorter version is that I walked those winding streets for hours and days and weeks and it filled me with words.

I would like to thank my miniature Australian shepherd, Coco, who became my walking companion in Utah as I tried to recreate the rhythm of Paris at Liberty Park in Salt Lake City.

This book would also not be possible were it not for the guidance and friendship and humanity of my dear friend Kelly Wickham who believed in me so fervently that I started to believe her. She was the first friend I told about the treatment before I started and without hesitation she responded with, "Hell, yeah!" I will never forget the confidence her voice communicated to me in those two words.

I want to thank Phantogram, War on Drugs, Rostam, Yoke Lore, Adorable, and Conner Youngblood for creating the soundtrack to my recovery.

Thanks to Jon Sponaas for bringing me alive for the first time, for reminding me what it meant to want to feel things. Thanks go to VJC for showing me that it was possible to fall in love again. Thanks to Joleen Willardsen for demanding I stay behind at a fundraiser so that I could have drinks with the man who would eventually facilitate every line and word and paragraph of this book. All my love and adoration and devotion to Pete Ashdown. He jumped over a table for me, fell into a pond to fetch my hat. He opened his home to me and the two girls whose needs and wants and bedtime routines kept me alive. I would not have been able to accept his support or his willingness to nurture my work were it not for this treatment. I will love him until the death of universes not yet born.

I want to thank my mother, Linda Oar, and my stepfather, Robert Oar. This entire book is a love letter to them both. They sacrificed their lives so that I might live, and I strive to be worthy of that gift every day. Their legacy will be all the amazing work done by people they have offered unwavering generosity, work made possible because they showed up again and again. Their legacy will be a generation of children who know how to love because they saw it modeled in their grandparents.

And finally, I want to thank the two girls who have inspired every word I have ever written. My life is a love letter to Leta Elise and Marlo Iris. I want to live to see them live. My love for them is what made me hold on, and my biggest hope in life is that I can be the mother to them that my mother has been to me.

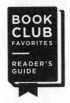

BOOK
CLUB
FAVORITES
—
READER'S
GUIDE

THE
VALEDICTORIAN
OF BEING
DEAD

HEATHER B.
ARMSTRONG

This reading group guide for The Valedictorian of Being Dead: The
True Story of Dying Ten Times to Live *includes an introduction,
discussion questions, and ideas for enhancing your book club. The suggested questions are intended to help your reading group find new and
interesting angles and topics for your discussion. We hope that these ideas
will enrich your conversation and increase your enjoyment of the book.*

INTRODUCTION

Heather B. Armstrong might be best known as the mommy blogger behind the incredibly popular website *dooce*, but she's also been struggling with depression all her life. A few years after her ex-husband moves across the country, Armstrong is drowning in depression, barely able to cope working full time and raising her two daughters as a single mom.

Desperate to clear the fog of depression, she agrees to a study that will take her close to brain death over and over again. It was possible the procedure could do nothing, but it was also possible it could reproduce the benefits of electroshock therapy without the side effects. Over the course of her treatment, Armstrong re-evaluates her relationships with family members, her kids, herself, and most important, her depression.

TOPICS & QUESTIONS FOR DISCUSSION

1. The title *The Valedictorian of Being Dead* comes from the book's prologue, in which author Heather B. Armstrong takes pride in how well she approximates being dead. In other parts of the memoir, she clearly relishes being the best at whatever she does. What do you think this says about Armstrong's personality? How might it play into her depression?

2. To those looking in from the outside, Armstrong was successfully managing being a single parent to two daughters while working full time. However, she was barely getting by on the inside. Have there been times when it seemed like you had it all together but were actually falling apart?

3. Armstrong is well known as a "mommy blogger." If you're a parent, do you have any favorite mommy blogs? Take turns recommending the blogs and websites you have found the most useful on your parenting journey.

4. Armstrong makes it clear that suicide is not a selfish act—depressed people think that living is selfish because those around them would be better off if they are gone. Can you think about a time a person's suicide (or attempted suicide) affected you, and did you feel it was a selfish act? Have you re-evaluated that feeling since reading Armstrong's book?

5. The relationship between Armstrong and her mother is a focal point of *The Valedictorian of Being Dead*. Does this mother-daughter relationship seem familiar, or is your relationship with your mother more contentious than Armstrong's is? Take some time to discuss the benefits and drawbacks of having such a close relationship with your mother.

6. When she's at her worst, Armstrong turns to her mother and is able to be completely honest with her about her feelings without fear of judgment. Do you have anyone who plays that role in your life?

7. Have you had friends or family members who suffered from depression? If so, take turns discussing your personal experience with this disease and how we can be more empathetic to those with this illness.

8. Armstrong resorts to drastic measures to deal with her depression in this book, and the responses from the people in her life vary greatly. Why do you think her siblings' reaction is so wildly different than her father's and stepmother's?

9. As Armstrong continues her sessions, she begins to feel joy again as the depression lifts. She describes days of just feel-

ing happy. Have you ever been aware of your happiness like that? If so, take turns describing when it happened and how it felt.

10. One thing that struck Armstrong deeply was that everyone involved in the study was donating their time; they weren't paid to be there. Have you ever been moved in the same way by people volunteering because they believe something can make a difference? Have you ever volunteered your time over the long term?

11. Armstrong blows up myths around platitudes nondepressed people tell people who suffer from depression: for example, just get up and exercise and you'll feel better. Armstrong turns this on its head by volunteering to assist someone running the Boston Marathon because of her depression, and it makes things even worse. What are some of the other myths about depression that Armstrong busts over the course of her memoir?

12. Anxiety is a constant companion throughout this book, and it will probably feel familiar to many readers, even if they don't suffer from depression. Can you remember a time when anxiety got the better of you and how you were able to cope?

13. While Armstrong's treatment has done wonders for her, it may not work forever. If you were in her shoes and began feeling the depression returning, would you subject yourself to the treatment again, knowing how difficult it was the first time around?

ENHANCE YOUR BOOK CLUB

1. Pair *The Valedictorian of Being Dead* with another memoir on depression, such as Allie Brosh's *Hyperbole and a Half*. Compare and contrast the way depression is portrayed in the two books.

2. Read some of Heather B. Armstrong's sponsored brand posts on her mommy blog, *dooce*. Discuss her choice to stop accepting this type of income and whether you would have made the same decision.

3. Armstrong has a previous memoir called *It Sucked and Then I Cried*, which is about the birth of her first child. Pair these two books together and discuss how the threads of depression from the first book tie into her second.

4. Episode 102 of Armstrong's podcast is called "Destigmatize," and it confronts the suicides of Anthony Bourdain and Kate Spade. Listen to the episode, and then have a discussion about how we can all help to destigmatize mental health issues.